MULTIPLE
CHOICE
QUESTIONS

Based on The Monthly Add-On Journal

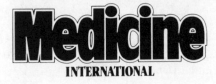

INTERNATIONAL

Prepared by a panel of London Consultant Physicians.
Foreword by William F. Jackson, MB, MRCP.
Editorial Director, MEDICINE International.

\STEST SERVICE
nel Hempstead
rtfordshire England

© 1984 PASTEST SERVICE
304 Galley Hill, Hemel Hempstead, Hertfordshire.

First published 1984

Reprinted 1986

ISBN 0-906896-15-0

British Library Cataloguing in Publication Data

Medicine international – Multiple choice questions.
1. Medicine – Problems, exercises, etc.
610'.76   R834.5

ISBN 0-906896-15-0

Phototypeset by Designed Publications Ltd, 8/10 Trafford Road, Alderley Edge, Cheshire. Printed by Martins Printing Works, Berwick-on-Tweed.

CONTENTS

Foreword   iv
Introduction   v
Examination Technique   vii
Medicine International   ix

INFECTIOUS DISEASES (65)   1

ENDOCRINE DISORDERS (16)   16

METABOLIC DISORDERS (26)   20

RHEUMATIC DISORDERS (30)   27

GASTRO-INTESTINAL DISORDERS (20)   35

LIVER DISEASE (20)   40

CARDIOVASCULAR DISORDERS (41)   45

RESPIRATORY DISORDERS (30)   55

BLOOD DISORDERS (24)   62

KIDNEY DISORDERS (30)   67

SKIN DISORDERS (15)   73

EYE AND EAR DISORDERS (12)   76

NERVOUS SYSTEM DISORDERS (41)   79

PSYCHIATRIC DISORDERS (15)   88

PREGNANCY AND PERINATAL LIFE (8)   91

AGE RELATED DISORDERS (7)   93

ANSWERS AND EXPLANATIONS   95

Brackets indicate the number of questions in each subject

FOREWORD

MEDICINE International, the monthly add-on journal, has been published in the UK since 1972, and the fifth series began publication in January 1984. The worldwide circulation of the English language editions of the journal approaches 250,000 copies per month, with a distribution covering 70 countries.

Multiple choice questions related to the content of the journal have appeared regularly since the beginning of the first series as an integral part of the journal. In addition, MEDICINE International has published a number of booklets containing further questions relating to the journal, which have been very well received. The questions are popular because they provide a painless and convenient method for the reader to test his knowledge of the content of the journal and, especially, because they closely parallel the kind of questions which appear in so many examinations — especially postgraduate diplomas such as the MRCP, MRCGP and their equivalents around the world.

Over the years we have made determined efforts to improve on the quality of multiple choice questions based on the journal. Our collaboration with PasTest has enabled us to produce questions of a consistently high standard and this second book contains a large selection of questions on all aspects of clinical internal medicine.

We hope that readers worldwide will find this book of value.

William F. Jackson MB MRCP
Editorial Director
MEDICINE International

INTRODUCTION

The aim of this book is to help the busy doctor test his medical knowledge in his occasional free moments or, if he is working for examinations, to enable him to revise in a methodical manner.

Systematic use of the book should indicate to the reader the subject areas in which he would benefit from further study.

HOW TO USE THIS BOOK

The book can be used on its own as there are brief explanations of the correct answers to all the questions. You will, however, obtain far more benefit from the book if you use it in association with MEDICINE International.

Each question is referenced to a particular issue and international page number in all editions of the first series of MEDICINE International.

These references are to be found in the answer section of this book from page 95 onwards. The information on pages x-xi will enable readers around the world to use the local edition of MEDICINE International for reference.

Your method of use of this book will depend on your educational needs and your personal preference. The questions can, of course, be used before and/or after reading the appropriate sections in the journal, and many readers find it helpful to 'pre-test' themselves before deciding upon necessary reading, subsequently 'post-testing' themselves.

Individual study:

● Do not attempt too many questions at one sitting -- in this way you are more likely to retain the new knowledge acquired.

● Limit yourself to one group of questions dealing with a specific topic -- this should help you to discover your weak points and enable you to use MEDICINE International to revise them.

● Try to avoid looking at the answers before making a definite decision with supporting arguments.

Group discussions:

This can be an effective way to use the book. Ask all participants to test themselves in advance on a set of self-assessment questions, and to study their answers in conjunction with the appropriate issues of MEDICINE International. Then discuss the answers with the other members of the group and make further reference to the journal if necessary.

MEDICINE International: you will get maximum value from these questions if you subscribe to MEDICINE International and read each issue as you receive it. The journal contains additional questions, not published in this book, relating to new material as it is published. Subscription details appear at the end of this book.

PASTEST: if you are working for examinations, other PasTest publications may be of great value to you. There are revision books and/or practice examinations available for those preparing for MRCP I & II, MRCGP, MRCOG, Primary FRCS and PLAB.

EXAMINATION TECHNIQUE

The multiple choice questions found in this book are based on the format used in many postgraduate examinations such as the MRCP I, MRCGP, MRCOG, Primary FRCS etc. Each question consists of an initial statement (or 'stem') followed by five possible completions (or 'items') identified by A,B,C,D,E. There is no restriction on the number of true or false items in a question. It is possible for all the items in a question to be true or for all to be false.

The four most important points of technique are:

(1) Read the question carefully and be sure you understand it.
(2) Mark your responses clearly, correctly and accurately.
(3) Use reasoning to work out answers, but if you do not know the answer and cannot work it out, indicate 'Dont Know'.
(4) The best way to obtain a good mark is to have as wide a knowledge as possible of the topics being tested in the examination.

To get the best value from this book you should arrive at an answer either 'True' or 'False' or 'Don't Know' for each item. Commit yourself before you look at the answer - this is really the best way to test your knowledge. In practice you can use the letters 'T', 'F' or 'D' to mark your answer against the question in the book. Alternatively you can prepare a grid on a separate piece of paper thus:-

	A	B	C	D	E
23					
24					

You can then mark your answers on the grid as you go along. To calculate your score give yourself (+1) for each correct item, (-1) for each incorrect item and zero for each 'Don't Know' answer.

All too often examination candidate's marks suffer through an inability to organize their time or through failure to read the instructions carefully. You must ruthlessly allocate your time. For example: in the MRCP Part I there are 60 questions to complete in 2½ hours, that is 2½ minutes per question or 10 questions in 25 minutes. Make sure that you are getting through the exam at this pace or a little quicker to allow time at the end for revision and a re-think on some questions you found difficult.

You must read the question (both stem and items) carefully. You should be quite clear that you know what you are being asked to do. Once you know this, you should indicate your responses by marking the paper bodly, correctly and clearly. In an official examination take great care not to mark the wrong boxes and think very carefully before making a mark on the computer answer sheet. Regard each item as being independent of every other item — each refers to a specific quantum of knowledge. The item (or the stem and the item taken together) make up a statement.

You are required to indicate whether you regard this statement as 'True' or 'False' and you are also able to indicate 'Don't Know'. Look only at a single statement when answering – disregard all the other statements presented in the question, they have nothing to do with the item you are concentrating on.

Since the answer sheets will be read by a computer they must be filled out in accordance with the instructions. As you go through the questions you can either mark your answers immediately on the answer sheet or mark them in the question book in the first instance, transferring them to the answer sheets at the end. In view of the time pressure you may be best advised to mark your answers on the answer sheets is you go along. Don't worry about marking the answer sheet very neatly the first time. Try to leave time to go over your answers again before the end, in particular going back over any difficult questions which you should have marked clearly in your question book. At the same time you can check that you have marked the answer sheet correctly.

Candidates are frequently uncertain whether or not to guess the answer. Experience shows that you should back your 'hunches'. Only if you are completely in the dark should you record a 'Don't Know' answer. Thus, if the question gives you a clue or your knowledge is sufficient to give you a 'hunch' about the correct answer, you will probably gain from guessing.

The answers and explanations in this book are necessarily brief, but they do provide a useful form of revision. The MEDICINE International references with each question give all the background information required to answer that question correctly.

MEDICINE INTERNATIONAL

References to further reading in MEDICINE International first series are given in the answer section of this book. Most page numbers are 'international' in that they are common to all editions of the journal.

A few numbers, however, are prefixed by a code letter specific to a particular edition. Such numbers indicate additional local material particularly relevant for readers of that edition, making the journal as relevant as possible to our readers in different countries.

Coding used in this book refers to three editions of the first series of MEDICINE International.

B   UK medical student and back number copies

M   Middle East

U   United Kingdom

The second series of MEDICINE International is being published in the following editions:

Australia	Starting April 1984
Indonesia (quarterly)	Starting March 1984
Pakistan (quarterly)	Starting March 1984
Southern Africa	Starting April 1984
The Far East (quarterly)	Starting March 1984
The Middle East	Starting January 1984
The United Kingdom	Starting January 1984

The 48 issues of the second series of MEDICINE International are published in chapters as follows:

1-3 Infections

4-5 Infection and tropical disease

6 Allergy and clinical immunology

7-8 Practical clinical pharmacology and therapeutics

9 Poisoning

10 Multisystem disorders and genetic disease

11-12 Endocrinology

13 Diabetes

14 Metabolic miscellany

15 Alcohol and disease

16-20 Cardiology

21-2 Rheumatology

23-6 Gastroenterology

27 Gastroenterology and liver disorders

28 Liver disorders

29 Oral medicine and sexually transmitted diseases

30-2 Renal disorders

33-6 Respiratory disorders

37 Critical care and emergency medicine

38-9 Oncology

40-1 Haematology

42-3 Dermatology

44-7 Neurology

48 Psychiatry

INFECTIOUS DISEASES

1. The human new-born infant

   A has received maternal IgM immunoglobulins by placental transfer in utero
   B has received maternal IgG by the same route
   C is protected against common infections for 6 to 12 months after birth
   D absorbs substantial amounts of IgA from colostrum if breast-fed
   E is unlikely to benefit from the administration of live vaccines before the age of 6 months

2. In passive immunisation

   A only IgG is transfered
   B resistance to infection lasts only three to four weeks
   C administration of human normal immunoglobulin gives reliable protection only against viral hepatitis type A and measles
   D human specific immunoglobulin is available for protection against viral hepatitis type B
   E protection against tetanus can only be obtained through the use of horse serum

3. Killed vaccines are used to provide protection against

   A measles
   B cholera
   C typhoid
   D pertussis
   E influenza

4. A boy of 10 is recovering from typical infectious mononucleosis with moderate splenic enlargement. The following considerations should determine his return to normal school activity:-

   A the Paul-Bunnell test must revert to negative
   B he should not play games as long as the spleen is still palpable
   C he is more likely to become depressed than is a girl of the same age
   D the patient's own sense of well-being is an unreliable guide to his actual degree of recovery
   E a prolonged and delayed recovery phase is less likely than in a man of 35

5. Paul-Bunnell-negative mononucleosis is a recognized finding in

    A   rubella
    B   herpes simplex
    C   viral hepatitis
    D   measles
    E   chicken-pox

6. The following are more often encountered in acquired cytomegalovirus infection than in infectious mononucleosis:-

    A   a typical lymphocytosis
    B   hepatic enlargement
    C   lymphadenopathy
    D   pharyngitis
    E   tonsillitis

7. *Toxoplasma gondii*

    A   is the most frequent cause of protozoal infection in England
    B   usually enters the human body via an infected water supply
    C   completes the sexual phase of its life cycle in the intestinal epithelium of the cat
    D   presents a small but definite risk to laboratory staff
    E   in human infections rarely causes clinical involvement of any site other than lymph nodes

8. Lassa fever

    A   usually presents as a continuous fever
    B   is most prevalent in rural areas of East Africa
    C   is thought to be mainly spread by droplet infection
    D   is a zoonosis affecting a small wild rat
    E   has not so far been transmitted from case to case in Britain

9. Chloroquine-resistant strains of malarial parasites have been detected as follows:-

    A   *P. falciparum* in South America
    B   *P. falciparum* in Kenya
    C   *P. vivax* in Pakistan
    D   *P. malariae* in Egypt
    E   *P. ovale* in Sri Lanka

10. A child who has just fallen ill and whose last contact with infectious diseases was 3 weeks ago might still be suffering from

   A   hepatitis A
   B   poliomyelitis
   C   rubella
   D   whooping cough
   E   chicken-pox

11. A child with one of the following infectious diseases is a potential source of infection at the times stated:-

   A   chicken-pox: five days before appearance of the rash
   B   mumps: five days before development of salivary gland swelling
   C   whooping cough: four weeks after the onset of symptoms
   D   measles: four days after the onset of the rash
   E   rubella: seven days before the onset of the rash

12. The following infectious diseases are statutorily notifiable in England and Wales:-

   A   tetanus
   B   ophthalmia neonatorum
   C   infectious mononucleosis
   D   infective jaundice
   E   syphilis

13. In the transmission of leprosy

   A   the usual source of contagion is a person suffering from the lepromatous form of the disease
   B   organisms from a human source are usually discharged from ulcer-ated areas of skin
   C   the number of viable bacilli released can be reduced to zero in a few weeks if rifampicin is administered
   D   susceptibility of individuals is determined essentially by the effectiveness of cell-mediated immunity
   E   lactating women with lepromatous leprosy are non-infective as long as lactation continues

14. Malaria prophylaxis is essential for travellers intending to visit

    A Japan
    B Sri Lanka
    C Central America
    D Cape Province, S. Africa
    E Algeria

15. *Wuchereria bancrofti* infection

    A is the most prevalent filarial disease affecting man
    B occurs commonly in tropical islands with a hot humid climate
    C is rarely found in urban communities
    D is transmitted by mosquitoes of the genus Mansonia
    E is maintained by reservoirs of infection in monkeys, cats and dogs

16. Recommended procedures for confirming the diagnosis of filariasis due to *W. bancrofti* include

    A lymph-node biopsy to demonstrate the adult worms
    B search for microfilariae in blood taken at the appropriate time of day or night
    C search for microfilariae in hydrocele fluid
    D examination of skin snips for microfilariae
    E testing for antibodies if no microfilariae can be found

17. In the treatment of infantile diarrhoea

    A antibodies have only a small part to play
    B the combination of atropine and diphenoxylate will give satisfactory results in the great majority of cases
    C the central problem is the restoration of normal fluid and electrolyte balance
    D oral glucose-electrolyte solution is usually effective replacement therapy
    E oral sucrose-electrolyte solution is usually effective in mild cases

18. Common causes of meningitis in the newborn include

    A *N. meningitidis*
    B *H. influenzae*
    C *E. coli*
    D group B streptococci
    E pneumococci

19. **Human filarial infections**

A   have a short natural life and so do not persist once the subject has left the endemic area
B   are transmitted only through mosquito bites
C   may be relatively innocuous
D   are diagnosed on the basis of the morphology of the adult worms
E   do not involve the multiplication of adult worms in the host

20. **In onchocerciasis** .

A   a short visit to an endemic area is unlikely to produce advanced lesions
B   the endemic areas are confined to Africa
C   the main pathology is due to the microfilariae rather than the adult worms
D   the skin rash is often itchy
E   involvement of the eyes may be confirmed by identifying the microfilariae in the cornea or anterior chamber

21. **Clinical manifestations of human toxocariasis include**

A   asthma
B   abdominal pain
C   iron-deficiency anaemia
D   retinal degeneration
E   cutaneous larva migrans

22. **When taking swabs for bacteriological investigation the following points are relevant:-**

A   results from dry swabs will be reliable as long as they are examined within 12 hours after collection
B   if a transport medium is used, examination within 24 hours will be satisfactory
C   if a dry infected area is swabbed the swab should first be moistened with sterile water
D   if tuberculosis is suspected, a specimen of pus should be sent rather than a swab
E   swabs of biopsy material are likely to be unsatisfactory

23. Unsatisfactory bacteriological results are likely if

    A a vaginal swab is sent for the isolation of *N. gonorrhoeae*
    B disinfectants are used in the collection of a mid-stream specimen of urine
    C venepuncture for blood culture is preceded by the use of potent agents to sterilise the skin
    D fluid from a suspected joint infection is refrigerated before being sent to the laboratory
    E urine specimens are refrigerated before being sent to the laboratory

24. The drug of choice for

    A Legionnaires' disease is erythromycin
    B meningococcal meningitis is sulphadiazine
    C prophylaxis of rheumatic fever is phenoxymethylpencillin
    D whooping cough is tetracycline
    E scrub typhus is carbenicillin

25. Treatment of leprosy should be guided by the following considerations:-

    A patients with the tuberculoid form should be isolated until the infection is brought under control
    B patients with the tuberculoid or borderline tuberculoid forms should be treated with triple therapy to prevent drug resistance
    C for orchitis due to leprosy the drug of choice is thalidomide
    D in the lepromatous or borderline lepromatous forms treatment should continue for the rest of the patient's life
    E type 1 lepra reactions should be treated with prednisone

26. Regarding diphtheria:

    A Diphtheritic myocarditis in those patients who survive recover completely with no subsequent cardiac disability.
    B If a palatal paralysis occurs and then recovers, full recovery from the illness can be confidently predicted.
    C Anterior nasal diphtheria carries almost no risk to the patient but is highly infectious.
    D Tonsillar diphtheria nearly always causes severe toxic symptoms and carries a very grave prognosis.
    E Skin diphtheria rarely causes other symptoms in the patient.

27. **Whooping cough**

   A is unusual in the newborn because of the protection afforded by maternal antibody
   B causes higher mortality among girls than among boys
   C has not yet been reported as causing death in a fully immunised child
   D is commoner in cold climates than in the tropics
   E is statutorily notifiable

28. **The following are characteristic clinical features of whooping cough:-**

   A fever during the catarrhal stage
   B tenacious sputum
   C vomiting
   D remission of coughing spasms as soon as the fever settles
   E conjunctivitis

29. **In the management of whooping cough**

   A neonates should always be admitted to hospital
   B antibiotics should be avoided in uncomplicated cases
   C if fits occur protection can be given with anticonvulsant drugs
   D coughing spasms can be prevented with anti-tussive drugs
   E during a spasm the child should be held in the head-up position to reduce congestion of the face and eyes

30. **In Rocky Mountain spotted fever**

   A the rash is usually petechial
   B CNS manifestations are unusual
   C serum from a convalescent patient usually agglutinates *Proteus vulgaris* (strains OX-2 or OX-19)
   D gangrene of fingers and toes may occur
   E a marked polymorph leucocytosis is characteristic

31. **The following are correct statements regarding the bacteriology of the abdomen and its contents:-**

   A In the colon, anaerobic organisms outnumber aerobic.
   B The renal pelves, ureters and bladder are usually sterile.
   C Liver abcesses are almost invariably caused by anaerobic organisms
   D The vaginal flora is exclusively aerobic.
   E *Bacteroides fragilis* is a common cause of salpingitis.

7

32. In the treatment of severe *Pseudomonas aeruginosa* infection, the following drugs are likely to be effective:-

A gentamicin
B tobramycin
C mecillinam
D mezlocillin
E ticarcillin

33. The following features are characteristic of the lepromatous rather than of the tuberculoid form of leprosy:-

A positive lepromin skin test
B numerous leprosy bacilli in affected sites
C erythema nodosum leprosum
D low or undetectable antibody levels
E amyloidosis

34. East African trypanosomiasis differs from the West African disease in the following respects:-

A The causative organisms can be clearly distinguished on morphological grounds from that causing the West African disease.
B The causative organism is more virulent to man than that causing the West African disease.
C Involvement of the nervous system occurs in East African but not in West African trypanosomiasis.
D The insect vector ranges widely through woodland areas, whereas that for West African trypanosomiasis is practically confined to waterways and their banks.
E A definite animal reservoir has been demonstrated, whereas none has been established conclusively for the West African disease.

35. In intestinal giardiasis

A symptoms when they occur usually begin within 48 hours of infection
B a symptomless carrier state is common
C trophozoites are unlikely to be found in the stools in the absence of diarrhoea
D trophozoites are an important source of infection
E patients should be told not to take alcohol while being treated with metronidazole

36. **The following are correct statements regarding *Entamoeba histolytica*:-**

    A   The establishment of *E. histolytica* in the human colon is usually symptomless.

    B   In the absence of diarrhoea, amoeboid forms (trophozoites) are not found in the stools.

    C   Amoebic dysentery, with bloody diarrhoea, usually causes fever up to 40°C.

    D   When the amoeboid form of *E. histolytica* is found in the stools of a patient with diarrhoea, this is reliable evidence that the diarrhoea is due to amoebiasis.

    E   *E. histolytica* alone is incapable of producing an inflammatory response in the human colon.

37. **In hepatic amoebiasis**

    A   the site most commonly involved is the left lobe of the liver

    B   there is normally a polymorph leucocytosis

    C   serological tests are positive in over 90% of cases

    D   most patients usually have diarrhoea

    E   metronidazole may be relied upon to effect a complete cure

38. **Important warnings that a patient may be suffering from falciparum malaria include the following:-**

    A   a regular pattern of fever every other day

    B   oliguria

    C   confusion

    D   jaundice

    E   constipation

39. **Advice as regards malaria prophylaxis should be based on the following principles:-**

    A   Antimalarial chemoprophylaxis should be started one week before travelling.

    B   Prophylaxis may safely be stopped one week after returning from a malarious area.

    C   For a short-term visit to a chloroquine-sensitive area, the best choice is pyrimethamine.

    D   If the patient is a pregnant female, the risk of teratogenesis from prophylactic drugs is more serious than the risk of malaria.

    E   Proguanil has a very low toxicity even when taken for many years.

40. In the collection of specimens for virological examination the following points are important guides to correct technique:-

   A   Viral transport media are more satisfactory than swabs as a means of transport to the laboratory.

   B   The optimum temperature for transport is 37°C

   C   The minimum rise in antibody titre which is acceptable as evidence of recent infection is four-fold.

   D   The best time for taking the second serum specimen for antibody detection is 2-3 weeks after the onset of the illness.

   E   The minimum acceptable sample of CSF for virological examination is 1 ml.

41. The following areas are free from rabies:-

   A   Denmark
   B   Australia
   C   Japan
   D   Ceylon
   E   United Kingdom

42. A man of 25 consults you on his return from a jungle expedition in South America during which (about six weeks previously) he was bitten by a vampire bat. He has no symptoms but is concerned about the risk of rabies. The following statements may be made:-

   A   In spite of the long period since the bite, the possibility remains that he could be incubating rabies.

   B   Infection with rabies can at this stage be proved or disproved by the estimation of rabies antibodies in the patient's serum.

   C   If there is a risk of rabies, protection can be given by the injection of human diploid cell strain vaccine.

   D   If the vaccine is to be given it should be supplemented by simultaneous injection of human rabies immunoglobulin.

   E   Once the virus has entered the peripheral nerves it is probably inaccessible to humoral defences.

43. **Primary tuberculosis**

   A   in developed countries is now commonly seen only in the pulmonary form
   B   is usually acquired from another patient with active pulmonary tuberculosis
   C   causes conversion of the tuberculin response to positive within one week after infection
   D   can usually be confirmed by the demonstration of tubercle bacilli in the sputum
   E   usually heals without complications

44. **Infection with coxsackie viruses may cause**

   A   epidemic myalgia (Bornholm disease)
   B   hand, foot and mouth disease
   C   myocarditis
   D   Japanese B encephalitis
   E   aseptic meningitis

45. **The use of griseofulvin should be guided by the following considerations:-**

   A   it is well absorbed from the gut
   B   to obtain the best results it is advisable to monitor serum levels of the drug
   C   no naturally resistant strains of dermatophytes have yet been found
   D   if it is given to a patient on anticoagulants without adjustments of the dose of the latter, there is a risk of spontaneous bleeding
   E   it has a potentiating action on the effect of alcohol

46. **The most reliable investigation for the diagnosis of**

   A   acute pulmonary histoplasmosis is the intradermal histoplasmin test
   B   chronic disseminated histoplasmosis is serology
   C   North American blastomycosis is culture of the organism
   D   invasive aspergillosis is repeated estimation of serum antibodies
   E   cryptococcosis is skin testing

47.   There is reliable evidence of a beneficial effect of

   A   amantidine in influenza A
   B   intravenous idoxuridine in herpes simplex encephalitis
   C   topical idoxuridine in herpes simplex eye infections
   D   intravenous vidarabine in herpes simplex encephalitis
   E   equine interferon in cytomegalovirus infection in transplant recipients

48.   The animal reservoir for

   A   yellow fever is monkeys
   B   dengue haemorrhagic fever is rats
   C   Marburg-Ebola virus fever is unknown
   D   Rift Valley fever is domestic animals
   E   Korean haemorrhagic fever is birds

49.   In human psittacosis

   A   the usual presentation is with a mild, influenza-like illness
   B   culture of the organism requires techniques appropriate to viruses
   C   a pneumonia is invariably present
   D   early treatment is essential if a long and debilitating illness is to be avoided
   E   the drug of choice is tetracycline

50.   Recognized manifestions of human *Brucella abortus* infection include

   A   depression
   B   conjunctivitis
   C   spondylitis
   D   polymorph leucocytosis
   E   lymphadenopathy

51.   Cutaneous anthrax

   A   usually occurs on exposed areas
   B   usually causes solitary 'malignant pustule'
   C   is extremely painful
   D   requires culture of the organism for bacteriological confirmation
   E   can be completely prevented in workers handling wool, hides and bonemeal by vaccination

52. **Orf**

    A   is primarily a disease of cattle
    B   in man is usually confined to the skin
    C   causes milkers' nodule
    D   should be treated with oral tetracycline
    E   is followed by a lasting immunity

53. **Leptospirosis**

    A   is responsible for up to 6% of all cases of lymphocytic meningitis in man
    B   can be confirmed by blood-culture in the first week
    C   can be confirmed by urine culture in the first week
    D   responds to treatment with penicillin
    E   in the home is usually acquired from infected cats

54. **False positive results from lipoidal tests for syphilis are known to occur in**

    A   malaria
    B   tuberculosis
    C   systemic lupus erythematosus
    D   viral pneumonia
    E   leptospirosis

55. **Recognized complications of non-specific urethritis in the male include**

    A   prostatitis
    B   epididymitis
    C   a generalized illness with fever and a pustular rash
    D   Reiter's syndrome
    E   proctitis

56. **Genital herpes**

    A   is caused by the same organism as lip herpes
    B   is often recurrent
    C   is usually transmitted sexually
    D   if uncomplicated will heal without treatment in about 10 days
    E   should be treated with penicillin if secondary infection develops

57. The following micro-organisms are capable of penetrating the placental barrier and infecting the fetus:-

    A *Staphylococcus aureus*
    B *Toxoplasma gondii*
    C Cytomegalovirus
    D Varicella-zoster virus
    E Hepatitis B virus

58. K-lymphocytes (Killer cells)

    A have surface receptors for Fc portions of 1gM molecules
    B require complement for their action on antibody-coated cells
    C play a part in renal homograft rejection
    D play a part in autoimmune thyroiditis
    E show characteristic morphological differences from T-cells and B-cells

59. HLA typing of the patient may provide important clinical hints in the diagnosis and management of

    A multiple sclerosis
    B ankylosing spondylitis
    C HBs-Ag positive hepatitis
    D myasthenia gravis
    E essential hypertension

60. In human leptospirosis

    A the clinical course is usually biphasic
    B if the organism is from the canicola serogroup meningitis may be a feature
    C a polymorph leucytosis is usual
    D blindness, if it occurs, is unlikely to recover
    E the drug of choice is penicillin

61. The rash of secondary syphilis

    A is first seen on the trunk and proximal parts of the limbs
    B is exclusively macular in character
    C spares the palms and the soles
    D is symmetrically distributed
    E occurs more profusely on extensor than on flexor surfaces

62. **Legionnaires' disease**

    A is normally acquired by infection from another case of the disease
    B in Europe and N. America is commoner in summer than in winter
    C appears to be a new disease, which did not occur before the American Legion convention in 1976
    D occurs in outbreaks having a positive association with modern hospitals and hotels
    E as seen in the U.K. is apparently acquired as a result of foreign travel in about one third of all cases

63. **Late syphilis**

    A is a term applied to manifestations of syphilis occurring five or more years after the initial infection
    B causing superficial lesions is non-infectious
    C may affect the tongue
    D can be relieved in all its manifestations by appropriate therapy
    E is a term not applicable to congenital syphilis

64. **Gonoccal pelvic infection in the female**

    A is commoner among women fitted with an intrauterine contraceptive device
    B is least common among women taking oral contraceptives
    C may be treated satisfactorily by an out-patient regime
    D can usually be diagnosed on clinical grounds alone without the need for bacteriological investigation
    E in doubtful cases may need to be confirmed by laparoscopy

65. **Definite laboratory confirmation of recent *Toxoplasma gondii* infection may be provided by**

    A a positive Paul-Bunnell test
    B a positive Sabin-Feldman dye test
    C the detection of specific IgM antibody
    D isolation of the parasite from the blood-stream
    E the passive haemagglutination test

66. **In the syndrome of inappropriate secretion of antidiuretic hormone**

    A   the majority of patients have no specific clinical features
    B   pulmonary oedema does not occur
    C   demeclocycline is effective through inhibition of ADH secretion
    D   lithium carbonate is more toxic than demeclocycline
    E   if the plasma sodium level falls to 110 mmol/l there is a risk of serious neurological manifestations such as fits or coma

67. **In the investigation and management of a patient with suspected Addison's disease**

    A   if the patient is ill, therapy with hydrocortisone hemisuccinate should be started immediately
    B   an abnormal short Synacthen test is not diagnostic
    C   maintenance on prednisolone or dexamethasone invalidates the Depot Synacthen test
    D   normal results for plasma electrolytes and urea rule out the condition
    E   adrenocortical antibodies are more likely to be found in a male patient than in a female

68. **In the investigation of a patient with suspected Cushing's syndrome**

    A   the most useful index of cortisol overproduction is the urinary free cortisol
    B   the serum γ-glutamyl transferase level may provide useful information
    C   a normal level of plasma ACTH at midnight makes the diagnosis of Cushing's disease very unlikely
    D   the metyrapone test is based on the power of the drug to supress ACTH production
    E   skull X-ray is of little value because of the small size of the tumour in Cushing's disease

69. **In the treatment of Cushing's syndrome**

    A   an optimistic attitude is justified in mild cases
    B   adrenal carcinoma recurring after surgery responds poorly to radiotherapy
    C   metyrapone may be helpful in Cushing's disease but not in other forms of the syndrome
    D   metyrapone treatment of Cushing's disease should be accompanied by steroid replacement, e.g. with dexamethasone
    E   the treatment of choice in Cushing's disease is bilateral adrenalectomy

70. Assay of the following hormones may be rendered unreliable if attention is not paid to the factors quoted:-

   A   angiotensin: posture
   B   thyroxin: recent ingestion of food
   C   growth hormone: anxiety
   D   prolactin: circadian rhythm
   E   aldosterone: diuretic therapy

71. In the treatment of hyperthyroidism with drugs

   A   the recurrence rate after stopping treatment is at least 50%
   B   satisfactory results can be obtained with a single daily dose of carbimazole or propylthiouracil once a euthyroid state has been produced
   C   propranolol must be given at least three times daily for continuous control of symptoms
   D   if a rash develops in a patient taking an antithyroid drug, treatment with all such drugs should be withdrawn permanently
   E   agranulocytosis developing in a patient taking an antithyroid drug will resolve within 1 - 2 weeks if the drug is withdrawn promptly

72. Treatment of hyperthyroidism with radioactive iodine

   A   takes 6 - 10 weeks to achieve a clinical response
   B   requires careful estimation of gland size to enable an exact dose of radioactivity to be given
   C   should not be given more than twice to any patient
   D   should be repeated if the patient has not become enthyroid within 4 months of the first dose
   E   carries no risk in adults of inducing leukaemia or thyroid cancer

73. In the interpretation of thyroid hormone assays it is important to remember that

   A   radio-immuno-assay of serum thyroxine measures all circulating thyroxine, both bound and free
   B   about 50% of circulating thyroxine is protein-bound
   C   no method is available for the direct measurement of thyroxine-binding globulin
   D   the 'free thyroxine index' is not a direct measurement of the free circulating thyroxine
   E   the T3 resin uptake test provides a measure of the circulating level of T3

74. Tri-iodothyronine (T3)

A is normally converted in the peripheral tissues to T4
B may be converted into reverse T3 (rT3)
C in T3-toxicosis is present at increased plasma levels because of preferential thyroid secretion
D in thyrotoxicosis is almost always elevated in the plasma
E in hypothyroidism is almost always depressed in the plasma

75. The use of progestogen-only oral contraceptives is governed by the following considerations:-

A ovulation is not regularly inhibited
B protection against pregnancy is as good as with the combined pill
C there is a substantial risk in older women of venous thrombosis and embolismm
D uterine bleeding may become irregular
E the dose of progestogen is much larger than in the combined pill

76. In the treatment of hypogonadism in the male

A adequate androgen replacement can only be achieved by parenteral administration
B patients with Klinefelter's syndrome tend to require more intensive therapy than those with other causes of testicular failure
C high-dosage androgen replacement may be complicated by macrocytic anaemia
D there is no known effective therapy for the eunuchoidism resulting from androgen resistance
E if secondary testicular failure is treated for long periods with androgens only it may be difficult or impossible to restore fertility at a later date with FSH injections

77. In the normal menstrual cycle

A the critical factor in promoting follicular maturation is a rise in pituitary FSH secretion
B increasing oestradiol secretion reduces the pituitary response to gonadotrophin-releasing hormone
C ovulation is preceded by a rise in pituitary secretion of LH
D after ovulation the corpus luteum secretes progesterone but not oestradiol
E the menstrual flow is preceded by a decline in progesterone secretion

78. The use of bromocriptine in the treatment of hyperprolactinaemia

   A reduces prolactin levels to normal in 95% of cases
   B is unlikely to restore normal menstruation if the condition has lasted longer than 3 years
   C may cause hypertension as a side effect
   D if successful results in reduction or abolition of galactorrhoea
   E is effective through its action on the hypothalamus

79. In a women whose sterility is thought to be due to Fallopian tube blockage:

   A if both tubes are blocked the outlook is hopeless
   B if patency is restored by surgery there is a high risk of a tubal pregnancy
   C extracorporeal fertilization offers an approximately even chance of success
   D tubal patency tests carry an appreciable morbidity
   E previous gonoccal infection may be responsible

80. In the treatment of dysfunctional hirsutism

   A cyproterone acetate acts by competing for androgen receptors
   B cyproterone acetate if given in high doses may cause excessive libido
   C a combined oral contraceptive will depress the levels of biologically active androgens no matter whether these are of ovarian or adrenal origin
   D if the androgens are of adrenal origin dexamethasone suppression will usually be effective
   E clinical improvement may be expected within 3 months

81. In Klinefelter's syndrome

   A the Karyotype is 47,XYY
   B spermatogenesis is normal in about one-third of the cases
   C plasma testosterone is undetectable
   D oestrogen levels are normal
   E FSH and LH levels rise markedly at puberty

82. In the interpretation of laboratory results in a case of hyperlipidaemia

 A accurate electrophoretic analysis is essential for a proper assessment
 B only fasting plasma samples are acceptable for diagnosis
 C a raised fasting plasma triglyceride with normal cholesterol indicates a rise in HDL
 D a raised fasting plasma cholesterol with normal triglyceride nearly always indicates a rise in LDL
 E a rise in the fasting plasma levels of both cholesterol and triglyceride is nearly always due to a combined rise in LDL and VLDL

83. In the clinical presentation of hyperlipidaemia

 A xanthoma tendinosum is virtually diagnostic of familial hypercholesterolaemia
 B attacks of pancreatitis are a manifestation of very high blood cholesterol levels
 C the finding of plantar or plamar xanthomas is consistent with the diagnosis of remnant removal disease (type III hyperlipoproteinaemia)
 D the elevation of plasma triglycerides associated with diabetes can be reversed by meticulous treatment of the diabetes
 E the hypertriglyceridaemia seen in diabetes and in chronic renal disease is associated with an increased risk of cardiovascular disease

84. A known diabetic is admitted with a provisional diagnosis of hyperglycaemic ketoacidosis. Your suspicions that the real diagnosis might be lactic acidosis would be increased if you found

 A an absence of hyperventilation
 B a negative plasma reaction to Ketostix
 C a history of treatment with chlorpropamide
 D a low blood pressure
 E a cold, clammy skin

85. Diabetic polyneuropathy

 A always produces well-defined symptoms
 B seldom causes motor weakness or wasting
 C is irreversible
 D is never associated with an autonomic neuropathy
 E affects the feet more often than the hands

86. **In heart disease in diabetics**

   A non-selective β-blocker drugs are preferable to selective β-blockers
   B treatment of hypertension with methyldopa may have undesirable consequences
   C high serum cholesterol levels should be treated in the first instance by dietary control
   D anaesthesia carries special risks
   E thiazide diuretics should be avoided

87. **In the assessment of diabetic control**

   A in well-controlled non-insulin dependent diabetes once-daily testing of urine is sufficient
   B glycosylated haemoglobin should be measured once a year to confirm the stability of control
   C haemolytic anaemia, blood loss and recent blood transfusion will cause falsely high values of glycosylated haemoglobin
   D in some types of haemoglobinopathy falsely low levels of glycosylated haemoglobin are found
   E estimation of·the reversible Schiff base precursor is superior to measurement of total glycosylated haemoglobin

88. **In the biochemical diagnosis of diabetes**

   A the two-hour blood sugar screen can give helpful indications but can never be diagnostic
   B a fasting venous whole blood glucose of 6.5 mmol/1 is diagnostic of diabetes regardless of the presence or absence of symptoms
   C if the fasting venous whole blood glucose is less than 7 mmol/1 but the two-hour value is between 7 and 10 mmol/1, the diagnosis of impaired glucose tolerance should be made
   D patients fulfilling the criteria of 'impaired glucose tolerance' must not be regarded as 'normals'
   E a pregnant woman fulfilling the criteria of 'impaired glucose tolerance' should be observed during pregnancy and re-assessed six months after delivery

89. In the case of a patient with non-insulin dependent diabetes treated with chlorpropamide in whom the ingestion of alcohol provokes a facial flush

   A a family history of NIDDM is more probable than in the case of a non-flusher
   B the risk of severe retinopathy is greater than in the case of a non-flusher
   C the risk of diabetic nethropathy is less than in the case of a non-flusher
   D it may be possible to block the response with aspirin
   E a small rise in acetaldehyde accompanies the flush

90. The development of symptoms in hypoglycaemia depends on the following considerations:-

   A the ability of brain tissue to metabolize ketone bodies gives substantial but transient protection against hypoglycaemia induced by excess insulin
   B adrenergic symptoms are most prominent when the blood glucose drops rapidly
   C insulin dependent diabetics of long standing tend to develop increasingly severe adrenergic responses to hypoglycaemia as their diabetes progresses
   D patients with insulinomas tend to have predominantly neurological rather than adrenergic responses to hypoglycaemia
   E short duration (1 - 2 hours) hypoglycaemia does not usually produce permanent neurological damage

91. Insulinoma

   A can usually be diagnosed by simultaneous plasma glucose and insulin determination
   B should be confirmed by measuring the blood glucose response to intravenous tolbutamide
   C is malignant in some 35 - 40% of cases
   D is relieved symptomatically by diazoxide in about 50% of cases
   E can usually be palpated at operation

92. Venepuncture was performed on a patient with 'difficult' veins by an incompetent operator who kept the cuff on for several minutes and repeatedly urged the patient to clench and unclench his hand. The serum sample so obtained did not show visible haemolysis. It might be expected to yield the following inaccurate results:-

    A   high serum protein
    B   high serum acid phosphatase
    C   high serumn creatine kinase
    D   low serum glucose
    E   low serum sodium

93. A blood sample from an elderly woman recovering from a fall shows an unexpectedly high serum alkaline phosphatase. The following should be considered as possible explanations:-

    A   undiagnosed fracture
    B   Paget's disease of bone
    C   prolonged exposure of the serum to sunlight
    D   history of alcoholism
    E   osteoporosis

94. In chronic lead poisoning

    A   diarrhoea is usually a prominent symptom
    B   in children convulsions may occur
    C   the diagnosis in suspected cases can be confirmed by measuring the serum lead level
    D   oral sodium-calcium edetate is effective therapy
    E   dimercaprol should be given by intramuscular injection

95. The following are correct statements regarding mercury poisoning:-

    A   metallic mercury in its liquid aggregate form is harmless if swallowed
    B   acute exposure to high concentrations of mercury vapour is likely to prove fatal within a few hours
    C   if a patient who has swallowed mercuric chloride survives the initial damage to the alimentary tract, uncomplicated recovery usually follows
    D   the treatment of choice for chronic poisoning is the administration of dimercaprol
    E   in the treatment of acute mercuric chloride poisoning, vigorous gastric aspiration should be the first step

96. A woman of 50 is admitted in coma; an empty bottle which is thought to have contained about 30 tablets, each of 25mg. imipramine, has been found by her bed. The following management decisions are correct:-

   A   she should be admitted to an intensive care unit
   B   gastric lavage should not be attempted
   C   the appearance of disturbances of rhythm on the ECG should be the signal for energetic treatment with anti-arrhythmic agents
   D   hypotension may respond to the administration of a plasma expander
   E   if the ECG shows no abnormality after 10 hours, monitoring can be safely discontinued

97. Fatal ventricular arrhythmias may result from the inhalation of

   A   petrol
   B   carbon tetrachloride
   C   trichloroethylene
   D   trichloromonofluoromethane
   E   dichlorotetrafluoroethane

98. Hallucinations may be caused by the ingestion of

   A   water hemlock (*Cicuta virosa*)
   B   deadly nightshade (*Atropa belladonna*)
   C   'greened' potatoes (*Solanum tuberosum*)
   D   death cap (*Amanita phalloides*)
   E   fly agaric *(Amanita muscaria)*

99. Osteoporosis may be a manifestation of

   A   Cushing's syndrome
   B   Klinefelter's syndrome
   C   alcoholism
   D   calcitonin-secreting tumours
   E   fluoride intoxication

100. **Recognized findings in malabsorptive osteomalacia include**

    A normal serum 25-hydroxy calciferol
    B proximal myopathy
    C raised serum alkaline phosphatase
    D 'codfish' vertebrae on X-ray of spine
    E therapeutic response to 1000 -2000 I.U. vitamin D daily

101. **In osteopetrosis of the recessive type**

    A symptoms usually first occur at puberty
    B the dense bones are unusually strong
    C anaemia is usual
    D thrombocytopenia may occur
    E there is excessive osteoclast activity

102. **In fibrous dysplasia of bone**

    A girls are more often affected than boys
    B precocious puberty is a recognized feature
    C the bone lesions are usually symmetrical
    D vitiligo is a common feature
    E the bones of the upper limbs are more often affected than those of the lower limbs

103. **Sodium excess may be a consequence of**

    A protein malnutrition
    B paralytic ileus
    C diabetes mellitus
    D hepatic cirrhosis
    E filariasis

104.   In hyperkalaemia

A   the patient's clinical symptoms and signs give ample warning that dangerous potassium levels are approaching
B   the ECG may show absence of P waves
C   a plasma potassium level greater than 6.5 mmol/1 is an indication for urgent treatment
D   the most immediately effective treatment is the oral administration of an ion-exchange resin
E   correction of alkalosis should be carried out as soon as possible

105.   Recognized causes of potassium deficiency include

A   intestinal obstruction
B   renal tubular acidosis
C   treatment with amiloride
D   malignant hypertension
E   carcinoma of the bronchus

106.   Undesirable effects in the control of diabetes may be caused by

A   phenylbutazone
B   chloroquine
C   propranolol
D   chloramphenicol
E   oestrogens

107.   In the management of snake-bite, apart from antivenom administration

A   heparin should not be used
B   morphine is valuable as an analgesic and sedative
C   freezing of the bitten area is a valuable emergency procedure which helps to delay dissemination of the venom
D   incision of the bitten area is usually unnecessary and may be harmful
E   immobilization of the bitten part, if possible, is effective in retarding venom movement

108.   In planning surgical treatment of rheumatoid arthritis

A   clinical evidence of nerve compression is an indication for priority treatment

B   if surgery is required for both upper and lower limbs the lower limb should be dealt with first

C   arthrodesis of the wrist produces such severe loss of function that it should only be performed as a last resort

D   arthroplasty is the first-line procedure for surgery on the rheumatoid wrist

E   rupture of a finger extensor tendon is best treated by simple suture of the two ends

109.   In the management of septic arthritis in a child

A   the most useful aid in early diagnosis is an X-ray of the joint

B   the drug of choice for antibiotic therapy in children aged 6 months to 2 years is ampicillin

C   surgical drainage should be the rule after an initial 24-hour period of antibiotic therapy

D   antibiotic therapy should be continued for 6 - 12 weeks

E   immobilization is necessary until the infection has been controlled

110.   A girl aged nine presents with a swollen painful right knee following a sore throat 10 days previously. The following considerations are relevant to the possible diagnosis of rheumatic fever:-

A   erythema nodosum would favour the diagnosis

B   in the absence of cardiac failure, a normal ESR rules out the diagnosis

C   a pericardial rub makes the diagnosis certain

D   subcutaneous nodules suggest that the correct diagnosis is almost certainly rheumatoid arthritis

E   a soft apical pan-systolic murmur favours the diagnosis of rheumatic endocarditis

111. **In Still's disease**

    A   the usual presentation is with an illness indistinguishable from adult rheumatoid arthritis
    B   the variety with polyarthritic onset is much commoner in girls than in boys
    C   about one third of affected children have anti-nuclear antibodies
    D   the presence of anti-nuclear antibodies in children with pauci-articular onset is closely associated with iridocyclitis
    E   rheumatoid factor is present in high titre in about 90% of cases

112. **In the management of juvenile chronic arthritis**

    A   an initial period of 2 to 3 months total bed rest will be beneficial in most cases
    B   swimming involves unacceptable hazards and should be forbidden
    C   aspirin is one of the drugs of first choice
    D   gold therapy is absolutely contra-indicated
    E   corticosteroids do not affect the ultimate prognosis

113. **Recognized findings in Henoch-Schonlein purpura in children include**

    A   an urticarial rash
    B   melaena
    C   a normal ESR
    D   abdominal pain
    E   increased level of IgA

114. **Nodules in rheumatoid arthritis**

    A   are found only in subcutaneous tissue
    B   imply an adverse prognosis
    C   occur almost exclusively in sero-positive patients
    D   occur over bony prominences at sites of pressure
    E   are found in less than 5% of cases

115. **Recognized findings in Felty's syndrome include**

    A   splenomegaly
    B   neutropenia
    C   thrombocytopenia
    D   leg ulcers
    E   lymphadenopathy

116.   The following considerations should govern the choice of anti-inflammatory drugs in rheumatic disorders:-

A   indomethacin carries a relatively high risk of peptic ulceration
B   salicylic acid preparations all require to be given at least 3 times daily
C   the propionic acid group of drugs has the lowest incidence of side-effects
D   the effectiveness of phenylbutazone in relieving the pain of ankylosing spondylitis constitutes a valuable diagnostic test
E   therapy should be planned so as to exploit the synergistic action of drugs from different chemical groups

117.   Treatment of arthritis with penicillamine

A   is ineffective in psoriatic arthropathy
B   must be withdrawn permanently if it produces a rash within the first month
C   if effective in rheumatoid arthritis causes improvement in extra-articular disease
D   is unlikely to succeed in patients with severe anatomical changes in the joints
E   must be monitored by full blood counts at least once a month

118.   In the treatment of arthritis, azathioprine

A   may cause neutropenia
B   is seldom of value in patients not responding to penicillamine
C   is valuable in progressive psoriatic arthropathy
D   may cause infertility
E   if the patient is receiving allopurinol, should be given in much increased dosage

119.   In the treatment of arthritis, chloroquine

A   is particularly valuable in arresting the progression of radiological change
B   is useful in cases of SLE
C   should be used with particular caution in patients over the age of 50
D   may cause a dose-related retinopathy
E   should not be given in a dose greater than 250 mg daily for more than one year

120. **Ankylosing spondylitis**

   A is less common in Negroes than in Caucasians
   B occurs in some 90% of all subjects carrying the HLA-B27 tissue antigen
   C is characterized by back pain which is least severe on waking and made worse by exercise
   D pursues a course in which attacks of pain are interspersed with relatively pain-free periods
   E may cause pain resembling that of pleurisy

121. **The arthritis associated with ulcerative colitis**

   A occurs almost exclusively in males
   B usually presents as a polyarthritis involving the wrists and fingers
   C can be abolished by total colectomy
   D usually causes no permanent damage to the joints
   E responds to intra-articular injection of steroids

122. **Arthrodesis is usually an undesirable procedure for arthritis**

   A in patients in the 20 - 30 age group
   B of the wrist
   C of the hip
   D of the metacarpophalangeal joint of the thumb
   E of the ankle

123. **Improvement following the therapy mentioned is to be expected in the arthropathy associated with the following diseases:-**

   A Whipple's disease: administration of penicillin
   B haemochromatosis: venesection
   C hypothyroidism: administration of thyroxine
   D familial Mediterranean fever: administration of corticosteroids
   E Fabry's disease: exclusion of cholesterol from the diet

124. **Characteristic features of mixed connective-tissue disease include**

   A myositis
   B cerebral disease
   C a better response to steroid therapy than in scleroderma
   D raised titre of DNA-binding antibodies
   E Raynaud's phenomenon

125. In systemic lupus erythematosus

    A evidence of renal involvement constitutes an indication for renal biopsy
    B the most specific diagnostic test is that for anti-nuclear antibodies
    C the best index of therapeutic response is given by serial immune complex estimations
    D the EEG is normal in the absence of overt cerebral disease
    E more than half the patients experience pleuritic chest pain

126. In polymyalgia rheumatica

    A symptoms are most severe on waking
    B there is usually a polymorph leucocytosis
    C muscular weakness is a striking feature
    D most cases resolve within 3 years
    E the illness may be a manifestation of occult malignancy

127. In the differential diagnosis between acute gonococcal arthritis and Reiter's syndrome

    A the presence of conjunctivitis rules out a gonococcal cause
    B gonococci can always be easily demonstated in gonococcal arthritis
    C fever over 39°C favours a gonococcal arthritis
    D a rapid response to appropriate antibiotic therapy favours gonococcal arthritis
    E the presence of tenosynovitis favours Reiter's syndrome

128. Characteristic findings in Paget's disease of bone include

    A raised serum alklaline phosphatase
    B decreased urinary hydroxyproline excretion
    C hypercalcaemia
    D decreased serum calcitonin levels
    E normal serum parathyroid hormone levels

129. **The following are correct statements regarding the treatment of soft tissue lesions:-**

A   a traumatic haematoma of the anterior thigh should be evacuated surgically as soon as possible because of the risk of myositis ossificans

B   complete rupture of a tendon requires prompt surgical repair for full recovery

C   sustained treatment of soft tissue lesions with non-steroidal anti-inflammatory drugs is of little value

D   continued activity after the development of a traumatic haematoma in muscle will greatly delay its resolution

E   a painful stiff shoulder should be treated with vigorous physiotherapy as early as possible

130. **A plain radiograph of the lumbar spine**

A   in osteoporosis will show diagnostic change when 25% of the bone mineral has been lost

B   will be normal in 25% of patients with disc prolapse

C   will show characteristic changes in at least 90% of patients with early ankylosing spondylitis

D   may show marked degenerative change in the absence of any symptoms

E   may show marked disc space changes in the absence of any symptoms

131. **The following clinical findings would make a diagnosis of prolapsed intervertebral disc unlikely:-**

A   absence of evidence of nerve root compression

B   evidence of compression of a single nerve root only

C   bilateral, symmetrical nerve involvement

D   pain which is unremitting

E   pain which is worse on resting at night

132. **The radiological appearances of osteoarthritis**

A   in the fingers are confined to the distal interphalangeal joints

B   in the cervical spine require posterior oblique views for their proper demonstration

C   in the first metatarsophalangeal joint may be confused with those of gout

D   in the knee are usually commonest in the lateral compartment

E   in the sacro-iliac joint characteristically include juxta-articular sclerosis

133. In the treatment of osteoarthritis

    A   swimming should be forbidden

    B   affecting the joints of one leg, a walking-stick if used should be carried in the hand on the same side as the affected joint

    C   if a walking-stick is used, it should strike the ground at the same time as the painful leg

    D   a walking-frame is a valuable aid for patients with arthritis in both legs

    E   drug therapy should be restricted to analgesics only

134. The following are correct statements with regard to the prevalence and epidemiology of hyperuricaemia:-

    A   serum uric acid concentrations are positively correlated with social class

    B   a serum uric acid concentration of more than 0.36 mmol/l (6 mg/100ml) in a male should be regarded as abnormal

    C   automated non-specific assay methods give results for serum uric acid which are on average 0.06 mmol/l (1 mg/100ml) lower than those obtained by a specific uricase method

    D   the commonest environmental cause for hyperuricaemia is the administration of diuretic drugs

    E   symptomless hyperuricaemia is some 20 times commoner than gouty arthritis

135. In the long term management of gout

    A   the drug of choice is allopurinol

    B   the patient should be advised to abstain from alcohol permanently

    C   probenecid should be avoided in patients with urolithiasis

    D   if allopurinol is to be used, administration should be started as soon as possible after an acute attack

    E   allopurinol therapy should be accompanied by a non-steroidal drug or colchicine for the first 3 months

136. The following are correct statements regarding immunological phenomena in rheumatoid arthritis:-

A   the antibody specificity of rheumatoid factors is directed against antigenic sites on the light chain of IgG

B   immunoglobulins with rheumatoid factor activity may belong to IgM, IgG and IgA classes

C   the expression 'rheumatoid factor' when unqualified always refers to IgM rheumatoid factor

D   immune complex formation and complement activation in synovial fluid have not been observed

E   synovial lymphoid cells in rheumatoid arthritis synthesize large amounts of immunoglobulin

137. The following are correct statements regarding laboratory tests for rheumatoid factor:-

A   the Latex test is sensitive but not very specific

B   the Rose-Waaler test is more highly specific but less sensitive than the Latex test

C   when IgM rheumatoid factors are absent (i.e. the patient is seronegative) IgG and IgA factors are absent also

D   nearly 100% of patients with Sjogren's syndrome are seropositive

E   the chance finding of a positive test for rheumatoid factor in an apparently normal patient indicates that overt rheumatoid arthritis is likely to develop in that patient within the next 5 years

138. Endoscopy of the upper gastro-intestinal tract

   A   is more effective than single contrast barium meal examination in identifying the source of a haemorrhage
   B   is essential in the management of gastric ulcer even if the radiological appearances suggest that the ulcer is benign
   C   in suspected peptic ulceration is unlikely to be of value if the barium meal is normal
   D   presents special hazards in patients with obstructive airways disease
   E   causing oesophageal perforation should be followed by conservative management

139. In allergic gastro-enteritis

   A   the pathological process is more marked in the stomach than elsewhere
   B   eosinophilia is characteristic
   C   in the small intestine there is villous hypertrophy
   D   serum IgE levels are raised
   E   macrocytic anaemia is usual

140. In the diagnosis of the acute abdomen, the finding quoted reliably excludes the condition listed with it:-

   A   a normal white cell count: appendicitis
   B   a normal serum amylase: acute pancreatitis
   C   absence of gas under the diaphragm in a plain X-ray of the abdomen: perforation of a hollow viscus
   D   absence of X-ray opacities in the gall-bladder area: gall-stones
   E   absence of fluid levels in erect X-rays of the abdomen: intestinal obstruction

141. Examination by barium meal X-ray

   A   should be followed by laxative administration for the two following nights
   B   may present special problems in the case of a patient with a phaeochromocytoma
   C   using single contrast technique may be expected to detect all but about 5% of lesions
   D   using double contrast technique is restricted to investigation of the stomach
   E   may be facilitated by the prior administration of cholinergic drugs

142. In gastric biopsy

  A intestinal metaplasia may indicate a predisposition to carcinoma
  B the scirrhous carcinoma of a 'leather-bottle' stomach is easy to recognize
  C peptic ulceration may produce changes which may be confused with those of carcinoma
  D infiltration of the lamina propria with inflammatory cells is a characteristic finding in atrophic gastritis
  E the appearances of superficial gastritis usually correlate well with the clinical findings

143. The following are correct statements about symptoms related to gas within the abdomen:-

  A belched wind is always air that has been swallowed
  B up to 2 litres of flatus per day may be produced by normal subjects
  C a diet high in pulses causes excessive gas production
  D carbon dioxide in flatus is mainly produced by bacterial action in the terminal ileum and large bowel
  E unless there is obvious subacute intestinal obstruction, borborygmi are always functional in origin

144. Recognized factors favouring the development of duodenal ulceration include

  A psychological stress
  B pregnancy
  C a positive family history
  D administration of steroid drugs
  E smoking

145. Following a six-week course of cimetidine in conventional doses, a patient with a duodenal ulcer still complains of typical ulcer pain. In this situation

  A endoscopy should be performed
  B the serum gastrin level should be measured
  C if the patient has an active ulcer, increased doses of cimetidine are unlikely to bring about improvement
  D a trial of colloidal bismuthate is worthwhile
  E surgery is unlikely to give a satisfactory result

146. **In the surgical treatment of peptic ulcer**

    A the operation of choice for uncomplicated duodenal ulcer is a Billroth II partial gastrectomy

    B the most widely-used procedure for gastric ulcer is a Billroth I partial gastrectomy

    C barium meal examination is unsatisfactory for the detection of post-operative recurrent ulceration

    D the patient's symptoms are usually a reliable guide in the diagnosis of post-operative recurrence

    E the first line of management in post-operative recurrence should be long-term cimetidine therapy

147. **A married woman of 26 is admitted to hospital with a history of melaena. On examination her pulse rate is 104 per minute and her blood pressure is 90/50 mm Hg. The blood haemoglobin is 13.0g/dl.**

    A The most urgent requirement in her case is to determine the site of the bleeding.

    B The absence of pallor indicates that the amount of blood lost so far is not serious.

    C A barium meal is not necessary if a skilled endoscopist is available.

    D If the haemorrhage is from a duodenal ulcer there is clear evidence that administration of cimetidine will have a beneficial influence on the outcome.

    E If surgery is to be undertaken, this should be delayed for at least three days after admission.

148. **A Meckel's diverticulum**

    A is commoner in males than in females

    B seldom causes bleeding in the elderly

    C may cause melaena

    D is best demonstrated by colonoscopy

    E should be excised if causing symptoms

149. **In patients with occult gastro-intestinal bleeding, the following skin conditions provide important possible clues as to the cause of the bleeding:-**

    A dermatitis herpetiformis

    B pseudoxanthoma elasticum

    C ascanthosis nigricans

    D psoriasis

    E neurofibromatosis

150. The following are correct statements regarding the processes of digestion and absorption:-

 A carbohydrates are absorbed into the mucosal cells in the form of monosaccharides
 B breakdown of carbohydrates to monosaccharides is completed by pancreatic amylase in the intestinal lumen
 C the function of bile salts is to act as carriers for fatty acids by forming complexes with them which are then absorbed
 D fatty acids finally enter the circulation in the form of triglycerides
 E absorption of small poeptides may be more efficient than that of the corresponding free amino-acids

151. A gluten-free diet aims at the exclusion of the proteins of

 A oats
 B wheat
 C barley
 D maize
 E rye

152. Antibiotics may be helpful in the treatment of

 A tropical sprue
 B Whipple's disease
 C intestinal lymphangiectasia
 D α-chain disease
 E systemic sclerosis

153. The following are significantly associated with oesophageal carcinoma:-

 A achalasia of the cardia
 B chronic iron deficiency
 C chronic lead poisoning
 D oesophageal caustic stricture
 E intestinal malabsorption

154. **Chronic intestinal ischaemia**

    A   causes lower abdominal pain after eating
    B   invariably causes loss of weight
    C   causes constipation but never diarrhoea
    D   is always due to atheroma of the arteries supplying the gut
    E   should be confirmed after clinical diagnosis by radio-active tracer measurements of intestinal blood flow

155. **In carcinoma of the colon**

    A   a palpable mass can be felt per abdomen in 50% of the patients
    B   estimation of carcinoembryonic antigen (CEA) is a valuable confirmatory test
    C   surgical treatment usually involves a permanent colostomy
    D   overall 5-year survival for patients treated in specialist units is about 50%
    E   if metastases do not develop within 3 years of diagnosis they probably will not develop at all

156. **In the management of Crohn's disease**

    A   surgical bypass procedures should be avoided
    B   the risk of ileal disease after pan-proctocolectomy is low
    C   the recurrence rate after segmental colonic resections is high
    D   in children, cortico-steroid therapy must be avoided at all costs
    E   serious clinical deterioration must be expected if the patient becomes pregnant

157. **In volvulus of the sigmoid colon in the elderly**

    A   idiopathic megacolon may be an antecedent cause
    B   there is usually associated diverticular disease
    C   pain is usually absent
    D   the colon is tender
    E   immediate laparotomy is the only safe procedure

158. **Endoscopic sphincterotomy for gall-stones in the common bile duct**

   A   is safer than surgery in elderly patients
   B   causes complications requiring surgical intervention in some 10% of cases
   C   carries an overall mortality of about 1%
   D   should only be used in patients who have already undergone cholecystectomy
   E   is contraindicated in the presence of pancreatitis

159. **In primary biliary cirrhosis, in addition to cholestasis, a 'dry gland' syndrome affects the**

   A   lacrimal glands
   B   mucus-secreting glands of the bronchi
   C   salivary glands
   D   pancreas
   E   sweat glands

160. **In the diagnosis of primary biliary cirrhosis**

   A   ERCP is hazardous and should be avoided
   B   a serum cholesterol level of more than 10 mmol/l (387 mg/100ml) indicates severe hepato-cellular damage
   C   accelerating hyperbilirubinaemia indicates a poor prognosis
   D   chronic pancreatitis can be demonstrated in roughly half the patients
   E   very high levels of serum aspartate transaminase are usual

161. **Hepatic involvement is common in**

   A   Felty's syndrome
   B   Still's disease
   C   systemic sclerosis
   D   cystic fibrosis
   E   primary amyloidosis

162. **The incidence of alcoholic cirrhosis**

   A   falls if the consumption of wine in the population falls
   B   is greater among doctors than among judges and lawyers
   C   is substantially reduced by heavy taxation on alcohol
   D   is greater in women than in men for a given alcohol intake
   E   depends on the amount of ethanol consumed rather than on non-alcoholic constituents of alcoholic drinks

163. **In the investigation of suspected acute pancreatitis**

A   a serum amylase level over 1875 IU/1 is diagnostic
B   a low serum calcium level indicates a poor prognosis
C   the presence of multiple fluid levels on abdominal X-ray is not uncommon
D   a milky serum indicates that a familial hyperlipaemia is the cause of the attack
E   methaemalbuminaemia indicates haemorrhagic pancreatitis

164. **In chronic pancreatitis**

A   if acute diabetes develops during an attack energetic treatment with insulin is essential
B   ERCP may show diagnostic changes
C   the serum amylase though seldom as high as in acute pancreatitis is always raised
D   fat necrosis is limited to intra-abdominal sites
E   pancreatic function tests are almost invariably abnormal

165. **In the investigation of a patient with suspected gall-stones**

A   plain X-ray will show the stones in some 50% of cases
B   CT scanning has greatly improved the detection rate
C   if the gall-bladder is not visualised on oral cholecystography a firm diagnosis of cystic duct obstruction can be made
D   cholescintigraphy may give useful information even in the presence of jaundice
E   in a non-functioning gall-bladder, stones may be detected by ultrasound

166. **Cholestatic jaundice is a recognized complication of treatment with**

A   ibuprofen
B   amitriptyline
C   iproniazid
D   propoxyphene
E   tetracycline

167. An alcoholic patient has developed tubercolosis and is to be treated with isoniazid and rifampicin. The following are correct statements:-

A   assessment of liver function before treatment is essential
B   monitoring of liver function tests is a valuable aid to management
C   if there is no evidence of liver damage within the first 3 months there will probably be none later
D   elevation of serum transiminase levels to not more than double the normal levels does not require immediate interruption of treatment
E   a rise in serum γ-glutamyl transferase requires immediate withdrawal of the drugs

168. In amoebic liver abscess

A   the onset is usually insidious
B   the presence of established cirrhosis makes the diagnosis unlikely
C   the quickest serological test is the cellulose acetate membrane precipitation test
D   the indirect haemagglutination test remains positive for years even after cure
E   the pus is normally odourless

169. In the management of ascites due to chronic liver disease

A   reduction of dietary sodium intake alone may be effective
B   treatment with diuretics requires hospital admission
C   the use of amiloride should be avoided
D   the presence of the non-A, non-B agent can be demonstrated by a rising titre of the specific antibody
E   therapy aimed at reducing portal hypertension is ineffective

170. In the diagnosis of viral hepatitis

A   the most reliable test for hepatitis A is the demonstration of virus in the faeces
B   the demonstration of HBsAg is a satisfactory way of diagnosing hepatitis B
C   the demonstration of HBeAg indicates that the patient is still infectious
D   the presence of the non-A, non-B agent can be demonstrated by a rising titre of the specific antibody
E   demonstration of HBcAg is of no diagnostic value

171. **Non-A non-B hepatitis**

    A rarely complicates blood transfusion
    B is often a subclinical infection
    C accounts for about 20% of viral hepatitis in developed countries
    D can be transmitted via infected drinking water
    E can be prevented in contacts with a high degree of certainty by the injection of human normal immunoglobulin

172. **In fulminant hepatic failure without previous liver disease**

    A if the patient survives the acute attack the long-term prognosis remains poor
    B the commonest cause is viral hepatitis
    C the bleeding tendency is mainly due to increased fibrinolysis
    D prophylactic administration of cimetidine almost completely prevents gastro-intestinal haemorrhage
    E respiratory alkalosis may develop in the early stages

173. **Characteristic findings in chronic persistent hepatitis include**

    A vascular spiders
    B splenomegaly
    C raised serum transaminase levels
    D raised serum IgG
    E progression to cirrhosis in some 25% of cases

174. **In the treatment of chronic active hepatitis type B**

    A bed rest is essential for the first 3 months
    B the intake of fat should be restricted to 20 g daily
    C aspirin should be avoided
    D corticosteroids should be given a trial in all patients
    E azathioprine should be given only in conjunction with prednisolone

175. **Liver biopsy is contra-indicated in the presence of**

    A prolongation of the prothrombin time by 5 seconds
    B a platelet count of $150 \times 10^9/l$
    C a haemoglobin level of 11g/dl
    D a suspected hydatid cyst
    E suspected primary hepatic carcinoma

176. Surgical removal of the following hepatic tumours is seldom possible:-

   A   cholangiocarcinoma
   B   angiosarcoma
   C   liver cell adenoma
   D   cavernous haemangioma
   E   focal nodular hyperplasia

177. In the control of bleeding in portal hypertension

   A   fresh blood is preferable to stored blood for transfusion
   B   if the patient has cirrhosis, the chances that the bleeding is from oesophageal varices are about 9 to 1
   C   vasopressin acts by reducing mesenteric and coeliac arterial blood flow
   D   the vasoconstrictor effect of vasopressin is restricted to the splanchnic circulation
   E   endoscopic injection is the most reliable procedure for the obliteration of gastric varices

178. In the clinical use of β-blocking drugs

A   a resting heart-rate of 40 beats per minute is an indication for withdrawal of the drug
B   drugs with partial agonist activity may be used in patients with heart failure
C   propranolol is valuable in the treatment of patients with airways obstruction
D   intermittent claudication may be made worse
E   nightmares and depression are particularly likely to occur in patients treated with atenolol

179. Once-daily dosage of the following β-blocking drugs is likely to be satisfactory:-

A   nadolol
B   oxprenolol
C   metoprolol
D   sotalol
E   alprenolol

180. Intravenous verapamil should not be given to patients who

A   have already received a β-blocking drug
B   exhibit signs of digitalis toxicity
C   have AV re-entrant tachycardia
D   have impaired sinus or AV node function
E   have hypertrophic cardiomyopathy

181. A patient being treated with digitalis runs a risk of developing digitalis toxicity if in addition he is given

A   amphotericin B
B   cholestyramine
C   nifedipine
D   quinidine
E   kaolin-pectin mixtures

182. Pre-systemic elimination ('first-pass metabolism') plays an important part in the pharmacodynamics of

   A   dextropropoxyphene
   B   digoxin
   C   imipramine
   D   propranolol
   E   chlorpromazine

183. The following features associated with pain the the chest are unusual when coronary artery disease is the cause:-

   A   occurrence following a heavy meal
   B   exacerbation by deep inspiration
   C   relief by sitting forward
   D   situation under left breast
   E   exacerbation by exposure to cold

184. 2-D echocardiography is superior to M-mode for

   A   assessment of left ventricular function in mitral regurgitation
   B   detection of organic tricuspid valve disease
   C   measurement of ventricular wall thickness in left ventricular hypertrophy
   D   detection of pericardial constriction
   E   detection of a left atrial myxoma

185. In aortic stenosis

   A   left ventricular enlargement is an early radiological sign
   B   there may be dilatation of the ascending aorta
   C   calcification of the aortic valve is almost invariable in patients over 40
   D   calcification and immobility of the valve are better assessed by echocardiography than by fluoroscopy
   E   bronchial arterial enhancement suggests that aortic valve replacement will soon be necessary

186. The radionuclide studies quoted are suitable for the investigation of the following cardiac problems:-

   A   measurement of myocardial perfusion: exercise thallium-201 myocardial imaging
   B   measurement of left-to-right shunt: intravenous injection of technetium-99m labelled microspheres
   C   myocardial infarction: uptake of potassium-42
   D   chamber filling sequence: first pass radionuclide angiogram
   E   ventricular function: radionuclide ventriculography

187. The following modes of treatment should be used with great caution in patients with the sick-sinus syndrome:-

   A   Digoxin
   B   β-blockade
   C   Verapamil
   D   carotid sinus massage
   E   DC shock

188. Accelerated idioventricular rhythm following acute myocardial infarction

   A   produces a broad QRS complex in the ECG
   B   persists continuously for many hours if not treated
   C   carries a grave prognosis
   D   may responmd to atropine
   E   may respond to lignocaine

189. Ventricular tachycardia

   A   may occur in the absence of any evidence of heart disease
   B   may be benign
   C   is always regular
   D   may be mimicked on the ECG by supraventricular tachycardia
   E   following myocardial infarction and occurring in episodes of 5 - 10 beats indicates that sustained tachycardia or ventricular fibrillation is very likely to follow

190. The ECG diagnosis of left bundle branch block would be supported by the finding of

A   an rSR pattern in the right precordial leads
B   a QRS axis of -40°
C   a deep S wave in lead 1
D   ST depression and T wave inversion in V5 and 6
E   prominent R waves in leads 1, V5 and V6

191. Vasodilator drugs are of proven efficacy in the treatment of

A   primary Raynaud's phenomenon
B   CRST syndrome
C   acrocyanosis
D   livedo reticularis
E   frost-bite

192. In the investigation of presumed deep venous thrombosis

A   venography involves a risk of pulmonary embolism
B   I-125 labelled fibrinogen yields results within a few minutes of its injection
C   ultrasonography may give false-negative results if the venous thrombosis is partially occlusive
D   impedance plethysmography is likely to give false-positive results
E   venography may be painful

193. Indications for pacing after anterior myocardial infarction include

A   complete heart block
B   RBBB with PFB
C   alternating RBBB/LBBB
D   isolated RBBB
E   isolated LBBB

194. A patient being prepared for open heart surgery should be told that

A   he may expect to leave hospital within 10 days if all goes well
B   he may expect to return to work within 2 - 3 months
C   if he is a Heavy Goods Vehicle driver. he may expect to resume driving within 6 months
D   he should avoid sexual activity after the operation
E   he should give up smoking

195. **Rheumatic fever**

    A   rarely follows streptococcal skin infections
    B   rarely occurs for the first time after the age of 15
    C   is some 2 to 3 times commoner in females than in males
    D   shows no evidence of genetic susceptibility
    E   is the commonest cause of heart disease in developing countries

196. **In an initial attack of acute rheumatic fever, the following signs favour the diagnosis of carditis:-**

    A   cardiomegaly developing during the attack
    B   gallop rhythm
    C   an aortic diastolic murmur
    D   an aortic systolic murmur
    E   tachycardia which is small in proportion to the fever

197. **In aortic stenosis**

    A   angina pectoris is commoner than in any other form of valve disease
    B   the murmur may be louder at the cardiac apex than at the base
    C   early enlargement of the cardiac X-ray shadow is characteristic
    D   calcification of the valve usually indicates a pre-existing lesion
    E   marked ECG changes constitute an indication for full cardiac investigation

198. **In mitral stenosis**

    A   the development of symptoms means that the valve area has been reduced to about 50% of normal
    B   recurrent bronchitis is due to raised bronchial venous pressure
    C   with regular rhythm systemic emboli are extremely rare
    D   anginal pain indicates coexistent coronary artery disease
    E   displacement of the apex beat indicates additional complicating cardio-vascular pathology

199.   Mitral incompetence may be a consequence of

   A   hypertrophic obstructive cardiomyopathy
   B   endomyocardial fibrosis
   C   systemic lupus erythematosus
   D   Klinefelter's syndrome
   E   pseudoxanthoma elasticum

200.   The implantation of a pacemaker

   A   may involve the risk of ventricular fibrillation
   B   requires a 'demand' unit in temporary pacing after acute myocardial infarction
   C   usually delivers an impulse to the right ventricle
   D   is known to prolong life in sinoatrial disorder
   E   is known to prolong life in chronic atrioventricular block

201.   Characteristic findings in infective endocarditis with aortic valve destruction include

   A   a wide pulse pressure
   B   displacement of the apex beat
   C   rapid development of cardiac failure
   D   left ventricular strain pattern in the ECG
   E   increased diameter of the cardiac shadow on chest X-ray

202.   Cyanosis first detected at the age of six months might be due to

   A   Fallot's tetralogy
   B   tricuspid atresia
   C   pulmonary atresia with intact ventricular septum
   D   double outlet right ventricle
   E   single ventricle with pulmonary stenosis

203.   Expected findings in ostium secundum defect include

   A   splitting of the second heart sound
   B   a pulmonary systolic murmur
   C   a pulmonary systolic thrill
   D   an rsR pattern in lead V_1 of the ECG
   E   development of heart failure before the age of 10

204. **Treatment with digoxin**

   A   is known to have a definite positive inotropic effect
   B   produces a diminishing response when given over a long period
   C   should be started with rapid loading with the drug
   D   requires larger doses for effective action in elderly patients
   E   is always preferable to the use of digitoxin or ouabain

205. **In the management of hypertrophic obstructive cardio-myopathy**

   A   the mainstay of treatment is β-adrenergic blockade
   B   the development of atrial fibrillation may produce spontaneous clinical improvement
   C   the use of verapamil should be avoided
   D   diuretics should be given routinely
   E   there is no place for digitalis therapy

206. **Heart failure is a common complication of**

   A   Hurler's syndrome (gargoylism)
   B   Friedreich's ataxia
   C   Duchenne muscular dystrophy
   D   facioscapulohumeral muscular dystrophy
   E   Pompe's disease

207. **Recognized findings in acute fibrinous pericarditis include**

   A   pain in the chest radiating to the left shoulder
   B   exacerbation of the pain on coughing
   C   atrial fibrillation
   D   depression of the ST segment in the ECG
   E   pathological Q waves in the ECG

208. **Cardiac tamponade may complicate pericarditis due to**

   A   tuberculosis
   B   uraemia
   C   malignancy
   D   rheumatic fever
   E   rheumatoid arthritis

209. **Dissecting aneurysm affecting the ascending aorta**

A   should be treated medically rather than surgically
B   may cause an aortic diastolic murmur
C   is best confirmed by CT scan with contrast enhancement
D   should not be investigated until the patient has recovered from the initial shock
E   should be treated initially with measures to restore the blood pressure

210. **In the investigation of a patient with hypertension**

A   a serum potassium below 3.5l mmol/1 is strongly suggestive of primary hyperaldosternonism
B   hyperuricaemia suggests a renal cause of the hypertension
C   intravenous urography should be carried out on all patients
D   ECG changes indicating left ventricular hypertrophy are useful predictors of complications of hypertension
E   CT scanning may be helpful in the diagnosis of phaeochromocytoma

211. **In acute myocardial infarction**

A   sublingual nitroglycerine does not relieve the pain
B   abnormal physical signs may be absent
C   bradycardia suggests anterior infarction
D   sinus tachycardia suggests that the infarction is a major one
E   pain may be absent in diabetic patients

212. **In the ECG after acute myocardial infarction**

A   the earliest change is ST depression over the affected area
B   reciprocal ST elevation is seen over the side of the heart opposite to the infarct
C   the pathological Q waves of transmural infarction are not usually seen until 72 hours or so after the infarction
D   persistent ST elevation and T wave flattening suggests the development of a ventricular aneurysm
E   in subendocardial infarction Q waves do not appear

213. **Cardiogenic shock in myocardial infarction**

A   is present if the systolic pressure falls below 90 mm Hg and there is evidence of poor tissue perfusion
B   when fully established carries a mortality of 90%
C   should be treated with inotropic agents
D   should not be treated with vasodilators
E   is usually accompanied by evidence of pulmonary venous congestion

214. **Exercise testing after proven or presumed myocardial infarction**

A   is safe provided that angina and cardiac failure are absent
B   is a valuable prognostic guide
C   is particularly desirable if the diagnosis of infarction is uncertain
D   allows valid conclusions only if the heart rate rises to at least 120 per minute
E   if normal indicates that the patient may return to a normal life

215. **Mortality following recovery from a myocardial infarct can be reduced by the long-term administration of**

A   timolol
B   aspirin
C   anticoagulants
D   sulphinpyrazone
E   disopyramide

216. **Recognized findings during an attack of stable angina pectoris include**

A   gallop rhythm
B   an apical systolic murmur
C   ventricular ectopic beats
D   ST segment elevation in the ECG
E   relief induced by caratoid sinus massage

217. **Medical treatment of a patient with acutely deteriorating angina pectoris should include**

A   β-blockade
B   ECG monitoring in a CCU
C   complete bed-rest
D   anticoagulant therapy
E   sedation

218. **Coronary artery spasm causing angina**

    A   is a very rare event
    B   is never fatal
    C   may occur in the absence of significant coronary arteriosclerosis
    D   should be treated energetically with β-blockers
    E   usually does not require surgical intervention

219. Cystic fibrosis

    A   occurs once in every 2000 births
    B   always causes a rise in sweat sodium level
    C   is due to defective production of the enzyme mucinhydrolase
    D   causes substantial pulmonary abnormality even before birth
    E   in the newborn commonly causes frequent loose stools

220. There is greater than average incidence in the U.K. of chest illnesses among

    A   infants whose parents smoke
    B   young chiildren in households where cooking is done by gas
    C   heterozygotes for α_1 -antitrypsin deficiency
    D   subjects living in large cities
    E   woodworkers

221. The following are reliable signs of hyper-inflation of the chest:

    A   increase in the PA diameter of the chest
    B   bilateral indrawing of intercostal spaces on inspiration
    C   reduction in the length of the trachea between the cricoid cartilage and the supra-sternal notch
    D   bilateral hyper-resonance on percussion
    E   absence of the normal cardiac dullness on percussion

222. In a patient with a restrictive defect of pulmonary function, the following results of lung function tests would be expected:

    A   normal FEV_1/FVC
    B   low PEF
    C   high TLC
    D   low lung compliance
    E   low transfer factor for carbon monoxide

223. Respiratory failure with a low PO_2 and a low PCO_2 in arterial blood is characteristic of

  A pulmonary oedema
  B pneumonia
  C bronchial asthma
  D pulmonary thromboembolism
  E chronic bronchitis with emphysema

224. In the treatment of respiratory failure

  A oxygen therapy should aim to produce a PaO_2 of at least 90mm Hg
  B oral nikethamide is a valuable long-term agent
  C doxapram is a safe agent with no hazard from over-dosage
  D tracheostomy should be avoided in chronic airflow obstruction if possible
  E venesection may be of value

225. There is clear evidence that the following modes of adjuvant therapy improve survival in patients with non-small-cell lung cancer treated surgically:-

  A immunostimulation by *Corynebacterium parvum*
  B pre-operative radiotherapy
  C post-operative radiotherapy
  D chemotherapy with methotrexate and cyclophosphamide
  E immunostimulation by levamisole

226. In the treatment of small-cell lung cancer

  A the response to chemotherapy is better than with other histological types
  B combinations of cytoxic drugs have not been shown to be superior to single drugs
  C radiotherapy plus chemotherapy is more effective than chemotherapy alone
  D the incidence of cerebral relapse can be reduced by radiotherapy
  E mortality from chemotherapy is unlikely to be less than 2%

227. **Primary pulmonary hypertension**

    A usually develops after the age of 50
    B is usually fatal within 8 years
    C may cause syncope
    D is not accompanied by cyanosis
    E shows a good initial response to treatment with pulmonary vasodilator drugs

228. **Primary infection with tuberculosis**

    A in the UK today is almost entirely airborne
    B can be prevented by the use of gauze masks
    C converts the tuberculin reaction to positive within 10 days
    D may remain dormant for many years
    E is always accompanied by bacteriaemia

229. **An anergic response to the tuberculin test occurs**

    A in sarcoidosis
    B in Hodgkin's disease
    C following infectious mononucleosis
    D following varicella
    E in immunosuppression

230. **The following anti-tuberculous drugs are bactericidal:-**

    A rifampicin
    B isoniazid
    C ethambutol
    D pyrazinamide
    E streptomycin

231. **Tuberculosis of the cervical lymph nodes**

    A causes tenderness of the affected node
    B in the U.K. is almost invariably due to *M. tubercolosis*
    C should be treated by chemotherapy for 6 months
    D should be treated surgically if rupture appears imminent
    E should be treated initially with a combination of three drugs

232. **In pneumonia due to *Str.pneumoniae***

A the disease caused by Type 3 organisms is particularly severe
B the organism is always sensitive to penicillin
C ampicillin is as effective as benzylpenicillin
D bacteriological diagnosis is impossible once treatment with antibiotics has been started
E failure of the X-ray appearances to resolve completely within 2 weeks strongly suggests an underlying carcinoma

233. **Tetracycline is effective in the treatment of pneumonia due to**

A *Klebsiella pneumoniae*
B *Legionella pneumophila*
C *Mycoplasma pneumoniae*
D *Chlamydia psittaci*
E *Coxiella burnetti*

234. **The following are characteristic clinical findings in acute extrinsic allergic alveolitis:-**

A wheezes
B obstructive-type respiratory defect
C raised $PaCo_2$
D onset of symptoms within 10-15 minutes of exposure
E persistence of radiological changes after clinical recovery

235. **The following are correct statements about extrinsic allergic alveolitis:-**

A farmer's lung is most prevalent during the hay-making season
B budgerigar fanciers have chronic rather than acute symptoms
C humidifier fever produces characteristic chest X-ray changes
D detergent lung is caused by products of *Bacillus subtilis*
E the aerodynamic size of the antigen particle must be less than $10\mu m$

236. **In the diagnosis of asthma**

A the contribution of skin tests is relatively unimportant
B reversibility by bronchodilators is a reliable diagnostic test
C paradoxical movement of the costal margin is not seen in large airways obstruction
D desensitization is an important mode of therapy
E sodium cromoglycate has no immediate bronchodilator effect

237. The following are correct statements about childhood asthma:-

    A   clinical asthma is not seen before the age of 2
    B   children with early onset of wheezing usually develop severe asthma
    C   asthma beginning in childhood nearly always persists into adult life
    D   chronic asthma is an important cause of short stature
    E   chronic asthma may cause delayed puberty

238. Essential investigations in childhood asthma include

    A   chest X-ray
    B   complete blood analysis
    C   skin tests
    D   IgE test
    E   radioallergosorbent test

239. Coalworker's pneumoconiosis with massive fibrosis

    A   is likely to progress even if exposure to coal dust is halted
    B   usually starts in the lower zones
    C   is commonly associated with bullous emphysema
    D   causes airways obstruction
    E   is more likely to occur when the coal dust contains a high proportion of silica

240. The following findings are consistent with the diseases mentioned:-

    A   favourable response to plasmapheresis: Goodpasture's syndrome
    B   phakoma: von Recklinghausen's disease
    C   lymphadenopathy and hepatosplenomegaly: Letterer-Siwe's disease
    D   exophthalmos: Hand-Schüller-Christian disease
    E   pneumothorax: tuberous sclerosis

241. In sarcoidosis

    A   an acute onset carries a bad prognosis
    B   the Kveim test is positive in about 70% of patients
    C   the serum angiotensin-converting enzyme test is highly specific
    D   the incidence is higher in whites than in blacks
    E   HLA studies have yielded conclusive evidence of a genetic factor

242. Respiratory function tests in cryptogenic fibrosing alveolitis characteristically show

 A normal FVC
 B reduced FEV_1
 C reduced lung volumes
 D reduced TCO
 E raised $PaCO_2$

243. In the management of cryptogenic fibrosing alveolitis

 A high doses of prednisolone occasionally produce a complete remission
 B respiratory function tests are a useful index of clinical progress
 C immunosuppressive drugs should not be used alone
 D penicillamine should be tried in all cases
 E a better prognosis can be given if the patient is male

244. In hydatid cyst of the lung

 A eosinophilia is nearly always present
 B calcification is usually seen on X-ray
 C the treatment of choice is surgical excision
 D the development of fever indicates that the cyst has become infected
 E the most reliable test is the indirect haemagglutination test

245. The finding of the following predominating in a pleural effusion would be consistent with the diagnosis mentioned:-

 A lymphocytes: malignancy
 B eosinophils: polyarteritis nodosa
 C multinucleated giant cells: rheumatoid disease
 D cholesterol crystals: obstruction of thoracic duct
 E mesothelial cells: pulmonary infarction

246. Characteristic findings in allergic bronchopulmonary aspergillosis (Type II) include

 A fever
 B airways obstruction
 C eosinophilia
 D mycotic abscesses
 E positive delayed haemorrhagic 'Arthus' response

247. **Characteristic features of asbestosis include**

    A   crackles heard at the lung bases
    B   wheezes
    C   clubbing of fingers
    D   increased incidence of lung cancer
    E   favourable response to steroid therapy

248. **Malignant mesothelioma**

    A   is particularly related to exposure to crocidolite
    B   is particularly increased among asbestos workers who smoke cigarettes
    C   usually presents with pleural effusion
    D   responds dramatially to radiotherapy
    E   requires tissue examination for its definite diagnosis

249. The following are correct statements concerning normally-occurring human haemoglobins:-

   A   the chain structure of Hb A is $\alpha_2 \beta_2$
   B   the chain structure of Hb F is $\alpha_2 S_2$
   C   a raised level of Hb F in adult life is virtually diagnostic of thalassaemia
   D   a defect in β-chain production involves only Hb A
   E   in children over 2, the proportion of Hb F is normally less than 3%

250. In the management of thalassaemia syndromes

   A   splenectomy is contra-indicated in β-thalassaemia major
   B   transfusion is unnecessary if the Hb remains above 9 g/dl
   C   a child with deletion of all four α genes may benefit from marrow transplantation
   D   small iron supplements are beneficial even if iron deficiency cannot be demonstrated
   E   in β-thalassaemia major normal growth and development can be achieved by an adequate transfusion programme

251. Antenatal diagnosis of the thalassaemia syndromes

   A   involves negligible fetal mortality
   B   is warranted if both parents have unequivocal β-thalassaemia minor
   C   requires amniocentesis only
   D   is justified if Hb H disease in the fetus is likely
   E   is contra-indicated if the fetus is likely to have the Hb Bart's syndrome

252. Iron is an essential component of

   A   cytochrome
   B   cytochrome oxidase
   C   catalese
   D   protoporphyrin III
   E   transferrin

253. The following are reliable indices of iron deficiency:-

   A   serum ferritin below $15 \mu g/l$
   B   MCHC below 30 g/dl
   C   MCH below 25 pg
   D   absence of stainable iron in a bone marrow biopsy
   E   raised free erythrocyte protoporphyrin

254. Reliable laboratory indices of early disseminated intravascular coagulation include

    A   increased fibrin degradation products
    B   prolonged prothrombin time
    C   positive ethanol gelation test
    D   prolonged thrombin clotting time
    E   positive protamine sulphate precipitation test

255. Increased size of the red blood cells can be caused by

    A   alcoholism
    B   gluten-sensitive enteropathy
    C   therapy with methotrexate
    D   heterozygous β-thalassaemia
    E   therapy with diphenylhydantoin

256. In pernicious anaemia

    A   patients with a family history present at an older age than those without
    B   antibodies to intrinsic factor are found only in patients with a family history
    C   bleeding from a peptic ulcer is a common cause of death
    D   jaundice is a recognized finding
    E   the serum level of vitamin B_{12} is always low

257. The following are consistent with a diagnosis of pernicious anaemia:-

    A   serum folate of 10μ g/l
    B   urinary excretion of 200 ng of B_{12} after an oral dose of $1\mu g$
    C   improvement of intestinal absorption of B_{12} when intrinsic factor is given
    D   plasma radioactivity of 0.1% of oral dose per litre at 12 hours ($1\mu g$ dose)
    E   failure of a patient to respond clinically to treatment with B_{12}

258. The following factors are believed to play a part in the pathogenesis of simple chronic anaemia:-

    A   shortened life-span of red blood cells
    B   impaired marrow response to anaemia
    C   failure of the reticulo-endothelial system to store iron
    D   defective transfer of iron to red blood cell precursors
    E   impaired transferrin production

259.   Secondary sideroblastic anaemia may be caused by

A   alcoholism
B   chronic active hepatitis
C   chronic arsenical poisoning
D   treatment with anti-tuberculous drugs
E   myeloproliferative disorders

260.   In the management of haemophilia

A   the analgesic of choice is aspirin
B   a haematoma in soft tissue requires urgent surgical decompression
C   prior to surgery the factor VIII or IX level should be raised to 30% of normal
D   factor VIII needs more frequent replacement than factor IX
E   hepatitis is no longer a hazard with modern cryo-precipitate

261.   A patient with a family history of haemophilia should be told that

A   the daughters of a haemophiliac have a 1 in 2 chance of being carriers
B   a carrier has a 1 in 4 chance of a haemophilic child at each pregnancy
C   the offspring of a carrier cannot be carriers
D   female relatives of haemophiliacs should have carrier detection studies
E   a family with mild haemophilia is unlikely to produce a severely affected child

262.   Treatment with methotrexate

A   does not produce acute toxic symptoms until 4-5 days after treatment
B   should never be used for long-term maintenance
C   frequently causes hepatic cirrhosis in patients with leukaemia
D   may cause pneumonitis
E   is less likely to produce toxic effects in the presence of ascites

263.   Thrombocytopenia is a well-recognized complication of

A   polyarteritis nodosa
B   hepatic cirrhosis
C   massive transfusion
D   Gram-negative septicaemia
E   treatment with chloramphenicol

264. The following are correct statements concerning blood platelets:-

    A   circulating platelets have no metabolic requirements
    B   some 30-40% of the total platelet mass is normally held in the spleen
    C   the half-life of circulating platelets is about 4 days
    D   there is a serious risk of intracranial haemorrhage if the count falls below 50×10^9 /1
    E   aspirin interferes with normal platelet function

265. In carrying out granulocyte transfusion it must be borne in mind that granulocytes

    A   from a leukaemic donor are accompanied by immature myeloid cells which may transmit leukaemia to the recipient
    B   carry ABO antigens
    C   carry HLA antigens
    D   if HLA incompatible will almost certainly provoke a reaction to the first transfusion
    E   separated by centrifugation are always contaminated with lymphocytes

266. In benign monoclonal gammopathy

    A   up to 15% of the bone marrow cells may be plasma cells
    B   the incidence of plasma-cell myeloma in the 10 years after diagnosis is less than 2%
    C   a normocytic anaemia is common
    D   there is increased susceptibility to viral infections
    E   soft-tissue plasma cell tumours are occasionally found

267. Recognized manifestations of macroglobulinaemia include

    A   epistaxis
    B   retinal haemorrhage
    C   lymphadenopathy
    D   hepatosplenomegaly
    E   nystagmus

268. The following drugs having haematological side-effects act through the mechanisms specified:-

    A   methyldopa: production of haemolytic auto-antibody
    B   methotrexate: interference with absorption of vitamin B_{12}
    C   aspirin: inhibition of thromboxane production by platelets
    D   cortisone: impairment of plasma-cell function
    E   sulphasalazine: oxidation of red-cell constituents

269. In a case of haemolytic anaemia, the following features would suggest that the haemolysis was intravascular rather than extravascular:-

   A   raised plasma methaemalbumin
   B   raised plasma lactic dehydrogenase
   C   absent plasma haptoglobin
   D   presence of haemosiderin in urinary deposit
   E   family history of favism

270. Meningeal leukaemia in children

   A   may be expected in over 75% of children with acute leukaemia if CNS prophylaxis is not given
   B   does not occur during haematological remission
   C   will not develop if CNS prophylaxis is given
   D   should be treated with intravenous methotrexate
   E   should always be treated with cranial irradiation

271. In the diagnosis of aplastic anaemia

   A   sparing of neutrophil polymorphs rules out the diagnosis
   B   a reticulocyte count of less than 0.1% of red cells indicates a poor prognosis
   C   no abnormal cells are seen in the peripheral blood
   D   bone marrow aspirate and trephine biopsy are both necessary
   E   isotope studies will often demonstrate extramedullary haemopoiesis

272. The following are correct statements about the Philadelphia chromosome in chronic granulocytic leukaemia:-

   A   if it is absent the prognosis is better
   B   it represents translocation of genetic material rather than loss
   C   it may be found in precursor cells of monocytes
   D   it is not found in lymphocytes
   E   it is responsible for the low neutrophil alkaline phosphatase

273. Haematuria

    A   in schistosomiasis is most marked at the start of micturition
    B   almost invariably accompanies proteinuria due to glomerular disease
    C   accompanied by a sore throat suggests mesangial IgA nephropathy
    D   of glomerular origin is always bright red in appearance
    E   may be caused by sickle cell trait

274. Interpretation of the plasma creatinine level may be subject to serious
      error in the presence of

    A   prolonged tourniquet time in blood sampling
    B   use of the wrong anticoagulant
    C   non-fasting status of the patient
    D   therapy with aspirin
    E   tubular secretion in renal failure

275. Dialysis is preferable to transplantation in the treatment of renal failure
      if in addition there is

    A   recent tuberculosis
    B   recent cancer
    C   chronic suppurative bronchiectasis
    D   severe uraemic osteodystrophy
    E   osteomyelitis

276. Patients on long-term dialysis must

    A   have a diet containing less than 0.5g protein per kg per day
    B   avoid added salt
    C   avoid occupations involving hard physical effort
    D   have specially purified water for the dialysis fluid
    E   avoid foods rich in potassium

277. Factors favouring the success of renal transplantation include

    A   original glomerulonephritis
    B   original analgesic nephropathy
    C   patient an American black
    D   blood transfusion
    E   youth

278. **In the management of chronic renal failure:-**

    A   urinary tract infection is best treated with co-trimoxazole
    B   protein intake should be restricted when the creatinine clearance falls
        below 10 ml/min
    C   dietary control of hyperlipidaemia is essential
    D   calcium supplements should not be given if there is severe hyperphos-
        phataemia
    E   the best calcium supplement is calcium carbonate

279. **adverse reactions to intravenous urography**

    A   usually occur within 5 - 10 minutes of the injection
    B   should be anticipated in patients with multiple myeloma
    C   if allergic in type, should be treated initially with an antihistamine
    D   can be prevented with certainty by prior administration of corticosteroids
    E   may include a generalized erythematous rash

280. **Recognized causes of macroscopic haematuria include**

    A   glomerulonephritis
    B   urinary tract infection
    C   accelerated hypertension
    D   renal cysts
    E   exposure to cold

281. **The following findings in a patient with renal failure suggest that the
     latter is terminal:-**

    A   Kussmaul respiration
    B   pruritus
    C   hiccough
    D   anaemia
    E   nocturia

282. **In Goodpasture's syndrome**

    A   the renal lesion is diffuse crescentic glomerulonephritis
    B   anaemia is unusual
    C   plasma exchange may be life-saving
    D   cyclophosphamide is contra-indicated
    E   about 40% of patients may be expected to recover

283. **Minimal lesion nephrotic syndrome**

    A   is the commonest cause of nephrotic syndrome in children
    B   usually occurs as a single episode only
    C   in children, should not be treated with steroids
    D   in adults, shows a 90-95% response to steroids
    E   seldom progresses to renal failure

284. **In the tropics, the following must be considered as possible causes of acute renal failure:-**

    A   *Plasmodium malariae* infection
    B   Typhoid fever
    C   *Schistosoma haematobium* infection
    D   Leptospirosis
    E   Sickle-cell disease

285. **In a hypovolaemic patient, the following would suggest that the renal hypoperfusion has progressed to renal tubular necrosis:-**

    A   urine volume 500 ml per day
    B   urine concentration 250 mOsm/kg
    C   urine sodium 50 mmol/l
    D   urine urea 200 mmol/l
    E   nephrogram on I.V.U. persisting for hours or days

286. **In Alport's syndrome**

    A   nerve deafness is invariably present
    B   women are usually less severely affected than men
    C   inheritance is autosomal recessive
    D   analysis of amniotic fluid allows antenatal diagnosis
    E   the disease does not recur in a transplanted kidney

287. **In adult polycystic disease of the kidney**

    A   renal enlargement is usually asymmetric
    B   the liver is not affected
    C   inheritance is autosomal dominant
    D   cerebral haemorrhage is a recognized complication
    E   there is an increased risk of malignancy

288. In the absence of treatment, death from chronic renal failure is the usual result of

   A   congenital nephrotic syndrome (Finnish type)
   B   adult polycystic disease of the kidney
   C   type I primary hyperoxaluria
   D   cystinosis
   E   familial recurrent haematuria

289. Recognized clinical manifestations of renal cell carcinoma (hypernephroma) include

   A   unexplained fever
   B   Budd-Chiari syndrome
   C   hypertension
   D   hypercalcaemia
   E   erythrocytosis

290. Alkalinization of the urine is an important measure in the prevention of the recurrence of

   A   uric acid stones
   B   triple phosphate stones
   C   cystine stones
   D   calcium oxalate stones
   E   methionine stones

291. The frequency of recurrence of calcium oxalate stones can be substantially reduced by means of

   A   use of water-softeners in hard water areas
   B   hydrochlorothiazide
   C   ascorbic acid in high dosage
   D   inorganic phosphate
   E   a milk-free diet

292. Renal biopsy may often yield unequivocal confirmation of the diagnosis of

   A   mixed connective tissue disease
   B   Henoch - Schonlein purpura
   C   amyloidosis
   D   thrombotic thrombocytopenic purpura
   E   Churg - Strauss polyarteritis

293.   Steroids and immunosuppressant drugs are known to be valuable in the treatment of the renal lesion in

    A   systemic lupus erythematosus
    B   polyarteritis nodosa
    C   Henoch - Schonlein purpura
    D   familial Mediterranean fever
    E   haemolytic-uraemic syndrome

294.   In the nephropathy of chronic hyperuricaemia

    A   the commonest histology is that of chronic interstitial nephritis
    B   a history of arthritis is often absent
    C   urate crystals are seldom seen in the renal cortex
    D   allopurinol may prevent further deterioration
    E   pyuria is usual

295.   Intravenous urography

    A   is the most useful investigation in the diagnosis of obstructive uropathy
    B   cannot be performed satisfactorily if the blood-urea is over 16 mmol/1
    C   should be avoided if there is renal failure due to diabetes
    D   in recent unilateral obstruction eventually yields a denser nephrogram on the affected side
    E   is a reliable guide to the size of the prostate gland

296.   In retroperitoneal fibrosis

    A   the aetiology is unknown in more than half the cases
    B   the ESR is usually normal
    C   corticosteroids are contra-indicated
    D   even after both ureters have been freed, long-term follow-up is needed
    E   bilateral ureterolysis is a major undertaking

297.   The following drugs should be used cautiously or not at all when the patient is in renal failure:-

    A   aspirin
    B   codeine
    C   morphine
    D   colchicine
    E   atenolol

298. In patients on dialysis, a dosage supplement of the following drugs is required to ensure adequate therapeutic levels:-

   A cloxaxillin
   B isoniazid
   C phenobarbitone
   D imipramine
   E allopurinol

299. **Analgesic nephropathy**

   A may be caused by paracetamol alone in therapeutic dosage
   B is more likely if paracetamol and aspirin are taken together
   C may improve if analgesics are withdrawn
   D may cause renal papillary necrosis
   E is associated with an increased incidence of ischaemic heart disease

300. **Covert bacteriuria**

   A in a pregnant woman should be treated expectantly
   B in a non-pregnant woman with a normal urinary tract requires no treatment
   C is virtually unknown in males
   D may contribute towards calculus formation
   E can always be demonstrated in the urethral syndrome of women

301. **Reflex nephropathy in the adult**

   A is diagnosed initially by intravenous urography
   B has a familial incidence
   C is commonly associated with analgesic nephropathy
   D is best treated by anti-reflux surgery
   E usually requires restriction of dietary salt intake

302. **Urinary tract infection in children**

   A in the first month of life, is commoner in males
   B is most likely to cause renal scarring when it occurs after the age of 2 years
   C accompanied by fever nearly always causes pyuria
   D accompanied by acidosis requires urgent intravenous urography
   E causes renal scarring only in the presence of vesico-ureteric reflux

303. The following dermatoses are pre-malignant:-

   A   solar elastosis
   B   solar keratosis
   C   Bowen's disease
   D   seborrhoeic keratosis
   E   Hutchinson's melanotic freckles

304. Koebner's phenomenon is a characteristic finding in

   A   pityriasis rosea
   B   psoriasis
   C   seborrhoeic eczema
   D   lichen planus
   E   warts

305. The following are recognized photo-sensitizing agents:-

   A   tetracyclines
   B   chlorpropamide
   C   frusemide
   D   chlorpromazine
   E   tar

306. In the treatment of skin disease with topical steroids

   A   clobetasol ointment involves little or no risk of systemic effects
   B   lesions on the face should never be treated in this way
   C   the therapeutic effect is enhanced by occlusion
   D   dilution by the manufacturer is preferable to dilution by the local pharmacy
   E   skin sensitivity may be caused

307. The following drugs may be effective in the treatment of acne:-

   A   ethinyloestradiol
   B   cyproterone acetate
   C   vitamin A
   D   prednisone
   E   co-trimoxazole

308. **Basal cell carcinoma**

A   regularly metastasizes to the regional lymph nodes
B   may occur in sites other than the face
C   is much commoner in men than in women
D   is resistant to radiotherapy
E   carries a grave prognosis even with energetic treatment

309. **Malignant melanoma**

A   in the UK is commoner in women than in men
B   always arises from a pre-existing benign melanocytic mole
C   is relatively insensitive to radiotherapy
D   has a nearly hopeless prognosis if metastases are already present
E   is best treated by cryosurgery in preference to excision

310. **Psoriasis**

A   is strongly associated with HLA type B17
B   is uncommon among American blacks
C   is virtually unknown before the age of 7 to 8 years
D   is characterized by an increased rate of epidermal proliferation
E   may be precipitated by bacterial infection

311. **The PUVA treatment for psoriasis**

Ingram : – dithranol plus tar bath then u.v. linght
U.VB used ie shorter wave length

A   takes longer than the Ingram regime to clear the rash
B   is safer than the Ingram regime
C   should not be used initially in patients under 50
D   is contra-indicated in pregnancy
E   involves some risk of hepatic damage

312. **Common contact skin sensitizers (as distinct from contact irritants) in developed countries include**

A   carbonless copy paper
B   lanolin
C   neomycin
D   industrial cutting fluids
E   epoxy resin

313. *Streptococcus pyogenes* is commonly the causative agent of

    A   erysipelas
    B   cellulitis
    C   bullous impetigo
    D   ecthyma
    E   Kaposi's varicelliform eruption

314. Herpes simplex

    A   is a common cause of erythema multiforme
    B   in the newborn is often fatal
    C   infection of the genitalia is always due to Type 2 virus
    D   primary infection is commonly followed by latent infection of sensory ganglion cells
    E   may cause permanent damage to the eye

315. Antihistamine therapy is often effective for

    A   symptomatic dermographism
    B   cholinergic urticaria
    C   cold urticaria
    D   pressure urticaria
    E   urticarial vasculitis

316. Cutaneous larva migrans

    A   is usually caused by *Strongyloides stercoralis*
    B   causes intense itching
    C   if not treated, persists indefinitely
    D   may cause a form of Loeffler's syndrome
    E   should be treated with thioguanine

317. In dermatitis herpetiformis

    A   men are more commonly affected than women
    B   no abnormal distribution of HLA factors has so far been found
    C   examination usually shows vesicles and bullae
    D   the response to dapsone is extremely variable
    E   a gluten-free diet may enable the dose of dapsone to be reduced

318. Recognized findings in acute anterior uveitis include

A   photophobia
B   dilatation of the pupil
C   keratic precipitates
D   a prolonged course lasting 6 months to 2 years
E   a good response to topical steroids

319. Retinitis due to the following organisms is an important hazard for patients undergoing treatment with immunosuppressive drugs:-

A   herpes simplex virus
B   herpes zoster virus
C   cytomegalovirus
D   Toxoplasma gondii
E   cryptococcus

320. **Chronic simple glaucoma**

A   is the commonest type of glaucoma
B   is commoner in whites than in blacks
C   is of unknown pathology
D   causes peripheral visual loss
E   should be diagnosed primarily on the basis of intraocular pressure measurements

321. **In chronic otitis media in childhood**

A   systemic antibiotics penetrate well to the middle ear
B   local antibiotic ear drops are nearly always effective
C   cholesteatoma is very uncommon
D   if the drum is perforated, swimming should be forbidden
E   removal of adenoids is beneficial whether they are enlarged or not

322. A positive Rinne test (air conduction better than bone conduction) would be consistent with deafness due to

A   old age
B   chronic otitis media
C   exposure to noise
D   streptomycin toxicity
E   tympanosclerosis

323. There is a recognized association between cataract and

    A   dystrophia myotonica
    B   injury to the eye
    C   chromosomal constitution 47,XXY
    D   primary hyperparathyroidism
    E   anorexia nervosa

324. In a patient presenting with corneal ulceration you would expect to find

    A   photophobia
    B   absence of spontaneous pain
    C   pain when light is shone into the unaffected eye
    D   flare
    E   green staining with fluorescein

325. CT scanning is superior to ultrasound in the diagnosis of the following orbital conditions:-

    A   exophthalmos due to thyroid disease
    B   meningioma
    C   dermoid cyst
    D   lymphoma
    E   lacrimal gland tumour

326. Cholesteatoma

    A   is a complication of chronic suppurative otitis media
    B   is an accumulation of cholesterol crystals in the middle ear
    C   may cause erosion of bone
    D   is a contraindication to mastoidectomy
    E   tends to recur after conservative treatment

327. In extrinsic rhinitis

    A   a muco-purulent discharge is characteristic
    B   desensitization is the treatment of choice
    C   topical steroids should be avoided because of their systemic effects
    D   sodium cromoglycate should not be used
    E   anti-histamines are undesirable

328. **In the diagnosis and management of squint in infancy**

 A   a family history of squint implies an increased risk
 B   correction of refractive errors may be curative
 C   corrective surgery at 6 months is much more effective than at 18 months
 D   corrective surgery after 2 years is relatively ineffective
 E   some degree of occlusion of the normal eye is essential

329. **Tinnitus**

 A   may be caused by disease in the external ear
 B   is always accompanied by some degree of deafness
 C   is much commoner in men than in women
 D   in Meniere's disease responds well to masking
 E   in depressed patients may be abolished by anti-depressants

NERVOUS SYSTEM DISORDERS

330. Following a head injury

A a period of unconsciousness unaccompanied by any other neurological abnormality represents functional change only without structural damage (concussion)

B the duration of post traumatic amnesia exceeds that of unconsciousness

C absence of any damage to scalp or skull is good evidence that no serious brain damage has occurred

D involving penetration of the skull, consciousness may be uninterrupted

E a fatal outcome is possible even if consciousness is fully regained with complete lucidity

331. Fracture of the skull

A is present in some 90% of patients with head injuries who develop intracranial haematoma

B can usually be excluded on clinical grounds without the need for an X-ray

C leads to intracranial infection in some 10% of cases of compound depressed fracture

D requires admission of the patient to hospital for at least 24 hours

E may lead to epilepsy five to six weeks afterwards but never before then

332. Late epilepsy after head injury

A develops in some 25% of patients admitted to hospital for head injury

B may not develop until 3 years or longer after the injury

C rarely involves focal manifestations

D is commoner in patients who develop early epilepsy

E is commoner in patients with depressed fracture of the skull

333. The following are correct statements about patients with head injury:-

A If coma lasts 6 hours or more, mortality will be about 50% regardless of details of management.

B If a patient regains the power of speech after the injury, a firm prediction of recovery can be made.

C If a depressed fracture of the skull has occurred, debridement and elevation must be carried out within 24 hours of admission to hospital.

B If the patient is unconscious on admission, an intravenous drip should be set up as soon as possible.

E patients with CSF rhinorrhoea remain at risk of meningitis for longer than those with CSF otorrhoea.

334. A man of 60 is referred with a provisional diagnosis of dementia due to Alzheimer's disease. Discovery, on examination, of the following would cast doubt on the original diagnosis:-

   A   inability to dress himself
   B   glabella tap reflex
   C   spastic weakness of one leg
   D   depression
   E   dysphagia

335. A previously healthy boy aged 15 months, during the course of a respiratory tract infection with a fever of 40°C (104F), has a generalized convulsion lasting 5 minutes.
   Initial management should include

   A   admission to hospital
   B   immersion in a bath at 0-1°C
   C   examination of CSF
   D   administration of aspirin
   E   administration of phenobarbitone

336. The following are helpful points in the recognition of classical petit mal:-

   A   absence of movements except of the eyelids
   B   provocation of an attack by hyperventilation
   C   normal intelligence
   D   seizures controlled without difficulty
   E   persistence of petit mal attacks into adult life

337. In the treatment of epilepsy with drugs

   A   a single daily dose of primidone can provide effective blood-levels throughout the 24 hours
   B   carbamazepine has a relatively short half-life and a single daily dose is not satisfactory
   C   phenobarbitone in correct dosage has no important side-effects
   D   phenytoin may cause hirsutism
   E   if phenytoin is to be given to a woman who is taking an oral contraceptive the dose of the latter must be reduced

338. **Drugs useful in status epilepticus include**

    A   intravenous diazepam
    B   intravenous phenytoin
    C   intramuscular phenobarbitone
    D   intravenous thiopentone
    E   intravenous imipramine

339. **Sodium valproate**

    A   is a drug of first choice for petit mal absences
    B   should not be used for petit mal with tonic-clonic seizures
    C   is likely to cause acne
    D   may cause alopecia
    E   should not be given to pregnant women

340. **In migrainous neuralgia**

    A   the attacks tend to occur at night
    B   men are more often affected than women
    C   the pain may last for up to 4-5 days
    D   a positive family history is usual
    E   a decrease in the plasma level of histamine is common

341. **In giant-cell arteritis**

    A   women are more often affected than men
    B   the diagnosis must always be confirmed by biopsy before treatment is started
    C   a pulsatile tender artery is better for biopsy than a non-pulsatile one
    D   oculomotor palsies do not occur
    E   treatment may have to be continued indefinitely

342. **The following are correct statements:-**

    A   Relief of compression in entrapment neuropathy always relieves the pain.
    B   Post-traumatic neuralgia may be relieved by sympathectomy.
    C   Surgical procedures for trigeminal neuralgia if effective inevitably cause anaesthesia of the affected area.
    D   Thalamic pain may take weeks or months to develop after a cerebral infarct.
    E   Relief after cordotomy seldom lasts longer than 2 years.

343. **Intracranial aneurysms**

A are multiple in about 15% of patients
B in the cavernous sinus usually produce clinical effects by rupture rather than through pressure on adjoining structures
C on the middle cerebral artery may cause intra-cerebral haemorrhage
D on the anterior communicating artery usually present with symptoms indicating pressure on the optic chiasma or nerve
E occur relatively rarely on the vertebro-basilar system

344. **Subarachnoid haemorrhage**

A when accompanied by an acute rise of blood pressure demands urgent measures to reduce the pressure to normal or below
B should not be investigated by lumbar puncture unless there is real doubt about the diagnosis
C usually causes xanthochromia of the CSF within 6 hours
D in patients over 65 should always be treated conservatively
E in patients under 50 with no abnormal neurological signs, normal blood pressure and normal CT scan requires no further investigation

345. **In the management of intracranial tumours**

A the best drug for the relief of headache is pentazocine
B biopsy is not always necessary
C radiotherapy has no beneficial effects on meningiomas
D with appropriate technique CT scanning can detect 95% of intracranial tumours
E EEG provides important diagnostic information in nearly all cases

346. **Hydrocephalus**

A in the great majority of cases is due to excessive production of CSF
B when described as communicating implies that CSF can pass freely from the ventricles into the subarachnoid space is a recognized manifestation of the Arnold-Chiari syndrome C
D may develop as a result of trauma
E has no hereditary basis

347. **Hydrocephalus is a recognized consequence of**

A tuberculous meningitis
B *H. influenzae* meningitis
C cocksackie virus meningitis
D toxoplasmosis
E toxocariasis

348. Recognized findings in normal pressure hydrocephalus include

    A   dementia
    B   disorientation
    C   unsteadiness of gait
    D   normal size of ventricles
    E   response to surgery for CSF diversion

349. In the diagnosis of hydrocephalus in children

    A   measurement of the skull circumference provides an absolute and independent criterion
    B   the occurrence of lid retraction is a misleading sign which should be ignored
    C   the skull X-ray may reveal the presence of abnormal bones
    D   the finding of intracranial calcification on X-ray suggests that haemorrhage from birth injury is the cause
    E   CT scanning allows accurate diagnosis without injection of radio-opaque material

350. In the diagnosis of hydrocephalus in adults

    A   a careful search should be made for evidence of intellectual deterioration
    B   papilloedema may be seen if the condition develops acutely
    C   CT scanning with injection of radio-opaque material allows the circulation of CSF to be studied
    D   thinning of the skull vault is one of the earliest radiological signs
    E   a previous history of subarachnoid haemorrhage is probably irrelevant

351. Shunt treatment of hydrocephalus

    A   is more satisfactory in children than in adults
    B   when complicated by infection regularly leads to high fever and marked constitutional disturbance
    C   may lead to the development of epilepsy
    D   in infants will inevitably require revision if the patient survives
    E   may cause a subdural haematoma

352.   In the case of a child admitted unconscious

    A   if tuberculous meningitis is suspected a CT scan must be done prior to lumber puncture
    B   the immunization history is important
    C   if non-accidental injury is the cause evidence of head injury will always be found
    D   if the onset is acute a neoplasm is unlikely
    E   if cerebral abscess is suspected, lumbar puncture is essential

353.   The following are correct statements about syphilis of the nervous system:-

    A   In tabes dorsalis *Treponema pallidum* can be demonstrated in the spinal cord.
    B   Lumbar puncture should be performed on all patients after completion of treatment for primary syphilis.
    C   The response to treatment of meningo-vascular syphilis is usually good.
    D   The course of tabes dorsalis is probably not affected by treatment.
    E   A Herxheimer reaction in the course of penicillin treatment should be treated with steroids.

354.   Multiple sclerosis

    A   is commoner in women than in men
    B   is very uncommon under the age of 10
    C   has an onset indicating multiple lesions in 80% of patients
    D   presenting with optic neuritis rarely causes persistent severe visual loss
    E   may cause trigeminal neuralgia indistinguishable from the idiopathic form

355.   Multiple sclerosis is likely to run a relatively benign course if

    A   onset is at an early age
    B   onset is with optic neuritis
    C   onset is with cerebellar lesions
    D   complete recovery from an episode occurs
    E   onset is with sensory symptoms

356. In the treatment of multiple sclerosis

   A   ACTH will shorten the duration of an acute relapse
   B   chronic treatment with ACTH will reduce the frequency of relapse
   C   oral steroids should be avoided
   D   the relapse rate can be reduced by intrathecal administration of interferon
   E   oral unsaturated fatty acids have no influence on the course of the disease

357. The following are correct statements about diseases of muscle:-

   A   Hypertrophy of calf muscles is seen only in Duchenne muscular dystrophy.
   B   Myotonia is not always present in dystrophia myotonica.
   C   Deep tendon reflexes are absent in most neuro-muscular diseases.
   D   Symmetrical muscular weakness usually indicates myopathic disease.
   E   Weakness following a heavy meal is suggestive of myasthenia gravis.

358. In the polymyositis/dermatomyositis complex

   A   well over half the cases are associated with carcinoma
   B   the initial weakness is usually of proximal muscles
   C   cardiac involvement does not occur
   D   steroid therapy is ineffective
   E   the best index of improvement is muscular strength

359. Characteristic features of malignant hyperpyrexia include

   A   autosomal dominant inheritance
   B   precipitation by exposure to halothane
   C   marked rise in body temperature within minutes of the onset
   D   cyanosis
   E   hypoventilation

360. The prognosis and management of Bell's palsy depend on the following considerations:-

   A   full recovery will occur spontaneously in about 95% of cases
   B   an incomplete palsy is a good prognostic sign
   C   in cases with incomplete recovery, some or all of the axons degenerate
   D   if the eye cannot be closed there is a serious risk of corneal ulceration and tarsorrhaphy is indicated
   E   there is now clear evidence that cortico-steroid therapy is effective in reducing the incidence and severity of denervation

361. Administration of thiamine is an important component of the treatment of

   A   alcoholic withdrawal seizures
   B   delirium tremens
   C   alcoholic cerebellar degeneration
   D   Wernicke's encephalopathy
   E   tobacco-alcohol amblyopia

362. The following are consistent with visual loss due to demyelination of one optic nerve:-

   A   a negative scotoma
   B   a larger pupil on the affected side
   C   Uhthoff's phenomenon
   D   pain on movement of the eyes
   E   impaired colour vision

363. Signs due to nerve root compression usually precede those due to compression of the cord in

   A   cervical spondylosis
   B   Paget's disease of a vertebral body
   C   spinal neurofibromatosis
   D   ependymoma
   E   epidural abscess

364. The Brown-Sequard syndrome includes

   A   spastic weakness on the same side below the lesion
   B   loss of proprioceptive sensation on the same side below the lesion
   C   loss of pain and temperature sensation on the opposite side below the lesion
   D   a lower motor neurone deficit in the myotome corresponding to the level of the lesion
   E   loss of light touch on both sides below the lesion

365. Myelography is an essential step in the diagnosis of

   A   motor neurone disease
   B   acute transverse myelopathy
   C   ependymoma
   D   epidural haematoma
   E   intradural meningioma

366. In the neuropathics complicating the following disorders, motor rather
      than sensory involvement usually predominates:-

      A   Guillain-Barre syndrome
      B   lead poisoning
      C   carcinoma of the lung
      D   uraemia
      E   diabetes mellitus

367. Essential tremor

      A   is absent at rest
      B   usually begins in the hands
      C   is made worse by even trivial amounts of alcohol
      D   does not respond to propranolol
      E   is made worse by stress

368. In Parkinson's disease

      A   progression of disease can be halted for several years by levodopa
      B   an association with HLA-B8 antigen has been demonstrated
      C   dementia does not occur
      D   a post-encephalitic origin should only be postulated if there is a clear
          history of encephalitis
      E   the commonest cause of death is pneumonia

369. The following are correct statements about anti-acetylcholine receptor
      antibody:-

      A   Reduction of serum antibody level by plasma exchange has been
          shown to produce transient clinical improvement in myasthenic
          patients.
      B   The antibody belongs to the IgM class of immunoglobulin.
      C   The antibody is specific to myasthenia gravis.
      D   Absence of a raised antibody titre rules out the diagnosis of myasthenia
          gravis.
      E   During clinical remission of myasthenia gravis the antibody becomes
          undetectable.

370. The following are characteristic clinical features of myasthenia gravis:-

      A   over 90% of cases suffer from diplopia or ptosis at some stage of their
          illness
      B   ocular symptoms are usually symmetrical
      C   muscular weakness is made worse by exercise
      D   the symptoms characteristically remit during pregnancy
      E   in a mild case, routine testing of muscular power may yield normal
          results

371. **Lithium carbonate**

   A   is ineffective during an episode of depression
   B   is ineffective in bipolar depression
   C   should not be given to elderly patients
   D   may cause severe anticholinergic side-effects
   E   when causing vomiting and diarrhoea should be withdrawn

372. **The following antidepressant drugs are effective when taken in a single daily dose:-**

   A   amitriptyline
   B   dothiepin
   C   viloxazine
   D   doxepin
   E   nortriptyline

373. **Schizophrenia**

   A   in western society is commonest in the lower socio-economic groups
   B   can now be positively identified by its characteristic biochemical abnormalities
   C   commonly causes auditory hallucinations
   D   is a frequent sequel of paranoia
   E   is very rare before puberty

374. **The prognosis in schizophrenia is relatively good if**

   A   the onset is acute
   B   there are no catatonic symptoms
   C   there is a known precipitating cause
   D   there are no affective symptoms
   E   there is no family history of schizophrenia

375. **Vivid dreams and nightmares are particularly common in patients being treated with**

   A   benzodiazepines
   B   propranolol
   C   methyldopa
   D   tricyclic antidepressants
   E   fenfluramine

88

376. Phobic anxiety

A occurs only in specific situations
B responds poorly to behaviour therapy
C is best treated by long-term therapy with benzodiazepine drugs
D may respond to tricyclic antidepressants
E requires special attention even if mild

377. Factors identified as important in increasing the probability of attempted suicide include

A lower socio-economic status
B divorce
C epilepsy
D residence in a rural area
E alcoholism

378. In the periodic syndrome

A poor parental discipline is often a cause
B the symptoms always disappear before the child becomes an adult
C pain at night is unusual
D the finding of similar symptoms in another member of the family suggest that the diagnosis is wrong
E drugs have no place in the treatment

379. Enuresis

A is technically defined as failure to develop bladder control by the age of 3 years
B is commoner among boys than among girls
C is commoner in the U.K. than in the U.S.A.
D is commoner in children of upper social class
E can seldom be shown to be due to a single cause

380. The following would favour a diagnosis of night terrors in a child rather than nightmares:-

A total lack of awareness of surroundings in an attack
B little or no amnesia for the episode
C marked autonomic disturbance
D association with REM sleep
E screaming

381. Doctors are more liable than the general population to

    A   hepatic cirrhosis
    B   suicide
    C   ischaemic heart disease
    D   schizophrenia
    E   depression

382. Oestrogen replacement therapy in menopausal women is more effective than a placebo in relieving

    A   depression
    B   insomnia
    C   poor memory
    D   anxiety
    E   palpitations

383. Prognosis is comparatively good for the following hysterical symptoms:-

    A   blindness
    B   vomiting
    C   fits
    D   inability to stand
    E   tremor

384. Disadvantages of the monoamine-oxidase inhibitors include

    A   poor control of anxiety
    B   delay of clinical response for up to 6 weeks after starting treatment
    C   pharmacological dependence if taken continuously for more than 1 year
    D   relative ineffectiveness in mild depression
    E   narrow spectrum of activity in neurotic disturbance

385. w-blocking drugs are particularly effective in relieving the following symptoms of anxiety:-

    A   palpitations
    B   nausea
    C   sweating
    D   flushing
    E   tremor

386. The following are correct statements about fetal breathing movements:-

   A They are absent for about ⅔rds of the time during the last trimester of a normal pregnancy.
   B Absence for more than 2 hours is a sure indication of fetal abnormality.
   C They decrease after maternal food intake.
   D They increase in the early morning.
   E They increase with the onset of labour.

387. In the management of pregnancy in a diabetic woman

   A admission to hospital for the last trimester is essential
   B routine delivery before 38 weeks is advisable
   C delivery should be by the vaginal route if possible
   D purified or human insulin is preferable to crude bovine or porcine preparations
   E monitoring of urinary glucose is unnecessary

388. The following drugs are known to be teratogenic in humans:-

   A diethyl-stilboestrol
   B chlorambucil
   C azathioprine
   D phenylbutazone
   E paracetamol

389. Respiratory distress syndrome of the newborn

   A is always obvious at birth when present
   B causes pathognomonic changes in the chest X-ray
   C is unusual in full-term babies
   D responds dramatically to supplementation of lung surfactants
   E should be treated routinely with antibiotics

390. A raised level of maternal serum α-fetoprotein may be due to

   A multiple pregnancy
   B threatened miscarriage
   C fetal neural tube defect
   D fetal abdominal wall defects
   E fetal kidney disorder

391. **Maternal mortality is significantly increased in the presence of**

   A   Marfan's syndrome
   B   valvular heart disease treated by curative surgery
   C   inoperable cyanotic congenital heart disease
   D   primary pulmonary hypertension
   E   congestive cardiomyopathy

392. **The baby of a diabetic mother runs**

   A   an increased risk of congenital heart disease
   B   a fivefold increase in risk of respiratory distress syndrome
   C   a 10% risk of developing diabetes
   D   a greatly increased risk of mental retardation
   E   a risk of hypomagnesaemia in the neonatal period

393. **Risk factors predisposing towards maternally transmitted neonatal infection include**

   A   prematurity
   B   female sex
   C   multiple pregnancy
   D   oligohydramnios
   E   previous reproductive loss

394. X-linked conditions causing childhood dementia include

   A   Fabry's disease
   B   ataxia telangiectasia
   C   Lesch-Nyhan syndrome
   D   adrenoleucodystrophy
   E   Tay-Sachs disease

395. Biotransformation of the following drugs is significantly slower in new-born babies than in adults:-

   A   phenobarbitone
   B   theophylline
   C   paracetamol
   D   nortriptyline
   E   phenytoin

396. Recognized changes in pharmacokinetics in the elderly include

   A   substantially decreased absorption from the gut
   B   decreased protein binding
   C   marked reduction in hepatic conjugation
   D   increased volume of distribution of fat-soluble drugs
   E   decreased volume of distribution of water-soluble drugs

397. Drugs known to cause confusion in the elderly include

   A   digitalis
   B   cimetidine
   C   quinidine
   D   methyl-dopa
   E   frusemide

398. Senile macular degeneration

   A   is commoner in men than in women
   B   is nearly always bilateral
   C   causes atrophy of choroidal blood vessels
   D   is mainly due to excessive exposure to ultra-violet light
   E   responds only partially to photocoagulation therapy

399. **Hypothermia in the elderly**

    A   is nearly always due to hypothyroidism
    B   usually causes tremor
    C   causes slow contraction and relaxation in the tendon reflexes
    D   if accompanied by hypotension is of severe degree
    E   usually causes hypercapnia

400. **Osteoporosis**

    A   is commoner in countries where the dietary intake of calcium is low
    B   in post-menopausal women is mainly due to increased bone resorption
    C   is commoner in obese subjects
    D   can cause loss of up to 65% of skeletal mass before radiological rarefaction of bone is apparent
    E   responds well to oral calcium therapy

ANSWERS AND EXPLANATIONS

The correct answer options are given against each question. The references given to MEDICINE International (1st series) and the issue numbers are in bold type. Almost all the references refer to the UK/International edition of the magazine, but where a page number is preceded by a letter (U11, B27) then this refers to a regional edition & material used for these questions has also appeared in the UK edition.

1. **B C E**   Ref: 1,15
   IgG is actively transferred across the placenta from mother to foetus but there is no such transfer of IgM or IgA. This maternal IgG has a half-life of 1 - 2 months in the baby and gives protection against common viral infections for 6 - 12 months; there is therefore no point in giving live vaccines before the age of 6 months. Colostrum contains IgA but this is not *absorbed* from the gut; its probable function is to protect against infections of the alimentary tract (eg. with enteroviruses).

2. **A C D**   Ref: 1,16
   In passive immunization the specific antibody transferred is entirely IgG. Its *half-life* in the recipient is 3 - 4 weeks and protection lasts *4 - 6* months. Human normal immunoglobulin, collected from unscreened pools of donor blood, contains effective amounts of antibody only for measles and hepatitis A.
   However, if the donors are screened for high antibody titre, sera can be prepared which are effective against hepatitis B and chicken-pox (human specific immunoglobulin). Human anti-tetanus and anti-rabies sera are now available.

3. **B C D E**   Ref: 1,16,17
   There is a trend towards the use of live avirulent vaccines but killed vaccines are still used against cholera, typhoid, pertussis and influenza.

4. **B E**   Ref: 1,34,35
   The Paul-Bunnell test in IM may remain positive for several months and the boy's own sense of well-being is a much more reliable guide to his actual recovery. However if the spleen is still palpable it is liable to be ruptured by external violence and games should therefore be forbidden. Depression would be a more likely sequel in a girl. The illness can be severe and prolonged in patients over 30; in younger patients this is less likely.

5. **A B C E**   Ref: 1,34
   Measles does not cause mononucleosis; all the other conditions mentioned may do so.

6.   B   Ref: 1,36
In acquired cytomegalovirus (CMV) infection atypical lymphocytosis is
less prominent than in IM and the Paul-Bunnell test is negative.
Lymphadenopathy, pharyngitis and tonsillitis are also less common than in
IM. However enlargement of the liver is relatively common.

7.   A C D E   Ref: 1,37
In England 30% of adults have serum antibodies to Toxoplasma and it is the
commonest protozoal infection., Human infection is acquired by eating raw
or undercooked meat containing the cysts of the parasite, or by ingesting
mature oocytes derived from cat faeces (the sexual phase occurs in the
intestinal epithelium of the cat). The lymph-nodes (usually cervical) are the
only sites commonly involved; the spleen is rarely palpable. Laboratory
infections may very rarely occur with strains of high virulence.

8.   A D E   Ref: 1,U12,B28
The continuous pyrexia of Lassa fever has occasionally caused confusion
with typhoid fever. The main focus is in West Africa.
Spread by droplet infection is now thought to be exceptional; the main risk is
from contact with blood, urine, secretion and other body fluids. The animal
host is a small wild rat, Mastomys natalensis. The infecting agent is a
member of the arenavirus group.

9.   A B   Ref: 1,6
All species of Plasmodium other than falciparum are sensitive to chloroquine
regardless of their country of origin. The main focus of chloroquine resistant
P. falciparum is in S.E.Asia, but cases have also been reported from
S.America and from Africa (Kenya and Tanzania).

10.   A B C E   Ref: 1.23
Incubation periods are as follows:-

Hepatitis A	2 - 6 weeks
Poliomyelitis	3 - 21 days
Rubella	14 - 21 days
Whooping cough	7 - 10 days
Chicken-pox	14 - 21 days

11.   A D E   Ref: 1,23
Periods of infectivity are as follows:-

Chicken pox	5 days before the rash to 6 days after the last crop
Mumps	3 days before salivary swelling to 7 days after
Whooping cough	7 days after exposure to 3 weeks after onset of symptoms

| Measles | From onset of prodromal symptoms to 4 days after the onset of the rash |
| Rubella | 7 days before onset of the rash to 4 days after |

12. **A B D**   Ref: 1,U11,B27
Infectious mononucleosis and syphilis are not notifiable: the rest are.

13. **A C D**   Ref: 1,9
In the tuberculoid form of leprosy the bacilli are very scanty and infection comes from cases with the lepromatous or borderline forms, in which the bacilli occur in large numbers in skin and the nasal mucosa; it is from the latter source that infection comes, since the skin organisms are not shed in significant numbers as long as the dermis remains intact. Rifampicin is bactericidal and renders such patients non-infective in a few weeks. Individuals with a good cell-mediated immune response either resist infection altogether or develop the tuberculoid form. Humoral antibody is produced in the lepromatous form, but is apparently ineffective. Lactating women with untreated lepromatous leprosy discharge large numbers of leprosy bacilli into the milk.

14. **B C E**   Ref: 2,U52
Malaria is a *tropical* disease; countries far enough north (e.g. Japan) and far enough south (e.g. southern extremity of Africa) are free from it.

15. **A B**   Ref: 2,78
Overpopulated tropical cities like Calcutta are heavily infested with *W. bancrofti.* The genus Mansonia transmits *Brugia malayi,* which unlike *W. bancrofti* is maintained by non-human animal reservoirs.

16. **B C E**   Ref: 2,79-81
Lymph node biopsy is *not* recommended because of the danger of producing lymph sinuses. For *W. bancrofti* microfilariae the blood sample should be taken as near midnight as possible.
Hydrocele fluid may contain microfilariae. *W. bancrofti* microfilariae are not found in skin: the skin-snip technique is appropriate for the demonstration of the microfilariae of Onchocerca volvulus.

17. **A C D E**   Ref: 2,54,55
Most cases of diarrhoea are viral rather than bacterial in origin, and even in bacterial cases antibiotics may favour the development of a carrier state. Atropine and diphenoxylate is a particularly dangerous combination which is absolutely contraindicated in infancy.

18. **C D**   Ref: 2,46
The organisms commonly responsible for meningitis in children and adults are relatively uncommon as a cause among the newborn.

19. **C E** Ref: 2,77

All the filariae for which man is the natural host are long- lived and may survive for up to 15 years. *Wuchereria bancrofti* filariasis is transmitted mainly by the mosquito *Culex fatigans* but other important filariases are transmitted by black-flies (*Onchocerca volvulus*) and horse-flies (Loa loa). Several human filariae, transmitted by midges, are relatively harmless. The diagnosis is based on the morphology of the microfilariae whihc are immature larval forms. These do not develop into adults in the same individual host and a heavy burden of adult worms is only aquired by repeated transmission.

20. **A C D E** Ref: 2,80

Severity of the disease is proportional to worm load and a heavy load requires prolonged exposure in an endemic area. Africa contains the main endemic areas but there are pockets in the Yemen, Mexico, Central and S. America. Slit lamp examination is essential for the diagnosis of ocular onchocerciasis.

21. **A B D** Ref: 2,65,74

Iron-eficiency anaemia is characteristic of hookworm infection (*Ancylostoma. duodenale*) and cutaneous larva migrans of infection with *Ancylostoma braziliense*.

22. **C D E** Ref: 3,93

Bacteria do not survive well on dry swabs, which must be examined within *4 hours* of collection if any confidence is to be placed in the results. Longer delay is permissible if a transport medium is used, but not more than *8 hours*. Bacteria from a dry area are protected to some extent from desiccation if the swab is moistened beforehand. Swabs from biopsy material are of little value; a piece of *unfixed* tissue should be sent in a sterile container.

23. **A B D** Ref: 3,95

Gonococci are fragile organisms and the vagina contains an abundant bacterial flora. The only satisfactory technique is to take *cervical* and *urethral* swabs and to culture these at once (the gonococci on the swab will die before they reach the laboratory). Disinfectants used in collecting mid-stream specimens may contaminate the urine and destroy the organisms being sought. Effective sterilisation of the skin before blood culture is essential to avoid contamination from skin organisms.

The organisms likely to be responsible for infections of joints, peritoneum or meninges are delicate and will be killed by refrigeration. In the case of urine, on the other hand, the longer the specimen remains at room temperature the greater the likelihood of bacterial growth (which will invalidate any attempt at quantifying the level of infection) and of degeneration of leucocytes and other cells.

24. **A C**   Ref: 3,98,99,134,U64
Erythromycin is effective in Legionnaires' disease and in mycoplasma pneumonia. The response of *N. meningitidis to* sulphonamides is variable and penicillin is now the drug of choice. Phenoxymethyl penicillin (penicillin V) is effective against *S. pyogenes,* can be given orally, is well tolerated and is inexpensive; no other agent compares with it for long term prophylaxis. In general, antibiotics have little effect on the course or duration of whooping cough; erythromycin may be of value very early in the catarrhal stage and may be useful if bronchopneumonia develops. The drug of choice for all rickettsial illnesses is chloramphenicol or a tetracycline.

25. **C D E**   Ref: 3,123,126
The lepromatous form constitutes a risk of infection to others, whereas the tuberculoid form does not. The recommended treatment for the latter is dapsone. Orchitis is a type 2 lepra reaction and for these thalidomide is the drug of choice. The initial therapy for the lepromatous form aims at rendering the patient non-infective with rifampicin; later dapsone should be given for the rest of the patient's life (depending on tolerance).

26. **A C E**   Ref: 3,110,111
Paralysis of the palate or of accommodation usually clears after a few days but this gives no guarantee that late (possibly fatal) paralyses of pharynx, respiratory muscles, limbs and cardiac nerves will not occur. Tonsillar diphtheria may be a relatively mild illness; the naso-pharyngeal form is much more serious and may be fatal within two weeks.

27. **B C D E**   Ref: 3,112
There is no protection from maternal antibody.

28. **A B C**   Ref: 3,112,113
The spasmodic stage persists long after the initial febrile phase and may last several weeks. The red eyes seen in whooping cough are caused not by conjunctivitis (more characteristic of measles) but by subconjunctival haemorrhages.

29. **A B C**   Ref: 3,113,-U64
Antibiotics are unnecessary unless bronchopneumonia has developed. Fits can be checked with intravenous diazepam or intramuscular paraldehyde and subsequently prevented with phenobarbitone or sodiumn valproate. Anti-tussives are ineffective. The main risk during a spasm is that of inhaling secretions or vomit, therefore the child should be turned head-down during the spasm.

30. **A C D**   Ref: 3,132-134
The initial lesions are maculo-papular but later almost always become petechial. CNS manifestations are common, including headache, restlessness,

confusion and (in severe cases) delirium.
A marked polymorph leucocytosis is unusual and suggestive of some complicating bacterial infection.

31. **A B E**   Ref: 3,114,115
Anaerobes such as *B. fragilis* are common causes of liver abscess but aerobic infections (eg. streptococcal) are also common. The vaginal flora is normally a mixture of aerobic and anaerobic organisms.

32. **A B D E**   Ref: 3,99,100
Gentamicin and tobramycin are effective against most strains of *P. aeruginosa;* a few strains are resistant and for these amikacin may be effective. Mecillinam is effective against many Gram-negative bacteria but not against *P. aeruginosa* or *H. influenzae.* Mezlocillin is a ureidonepenicillin active against *P. aeruginosa, B. fragilis* and *S. faecalis.* Azlocillin is even more effective against *P. aeruginosa.* Ticarcillin resembles carbenicillin: both are active against *P. aeruginosa* when given in high doses intravenously.

33. **B C E**   Ref: 3,123
In the lepromatous form cell-mediated immunity is not expressed but humoral immunity is (high antibody levels). Hence the skin test is negative, but immune complex disease may cause erythema nodosum and other lesions such as iritis, neuritis, orchitis, lymphadenitis or myositis. This humoral immunity is relatively ineffective and bacilli are abundant. Long-contained antibody production may lead to amyloidosis.

34. **B D E**   Ref: 4,162,163
T. brucei rhodesiense (E.African) is morphologically identical to *T. brucei* gambiense (W.African) but merits separate subspecie status because of differences in biological behaviour. Both organisms commonly invade the nervous system in man. The animal reservoir for gambiense is the ungulate population, particularly bushbuck; for rhodiense several reservoirs are suspected but none has been established conclusively.

35. **B C E**   Ref: 4,155-158
The incubation is usually about 8 days and may be over 2 weeks. Trophozoites are seldom found in formed stools but are frequently found in diarrhoeal stools. When passed in the stools they rapidly die and cysts are the only source of infection.

36. **A B E**   Ref: 4,159.160
E. histolytica in the human colon is usually harmless and non-invasive. Even when the invasion of the gut wall occurs it may be so mild as to cause no symptoms. In a normally functioning colon the absorption of water from the contents causes the amoebae to encyst; consequently formed stools contain cysts but no amoeboid forms. In a patient with symptomless

amoebiasis, any intercurrent cause of diarrhoea will prevent the encystment of the amoebae; hence the finding of amoeboid forms is not reliable evidence that amoebiasis is the cause of diarrhoea.

Amoebic dysentery usually causes little or no constitutional disturbance; high fever is more suggestive of bacillary dysentery. The inflammatory mass known as amoeboma is thought to be the consequence of some other factor in addition to amoebiasis, possibly low-grade infection with intestinal bacteria.

37.　B C　　　　　　　　　　　　Ref: 4,161

The commonest site is the right lower lobe. Concomitant diarrhoea is relatively rare. Treatment with metronidazole should be followed by a course of diloxanide furoate to eliminate the co-existent gut infection.

38.　B C D　　　　　　　　　　　Ref: 4,153

In falciparum malaria the fever is of irregular periodicity and often occurs daily; fever every other day suggests infection with *P. vivax* or *P. ovale*. Oliguria in falciparum malaria may be the prelude to acute renal failure. Confusion indicates that cerebral complications are imminent and jaundice may presage hepatic failure. Watery diarrhoea sometimes resembling that of cholera, is an uncommon complication of falciparum malaria.

39.　A E　　　　　　　　　　　　Ref: 4,154-156

Strictly speaking, if the first dose is taken the day before departure, prophylaxis will be effective. However most authorities recommend starting a week earlier, in order to detect any adverse reaction to the drug. Prophylaxis should continue for four weeks after leaving the malarious area. Chloroquine would be a better choice than pyrimethamine, which (being tasteless) may cause accidental poisoning and to which resistance may develop. There is no evidence so far of terato-genicity with chloroquine or pyrimethamine. Proguanil is recommended for long-term (3 years or over) prophylaxis.

40.　A C D E　　　　　　　　　　Ref: 4,135

Viral transport media provide optimum conditions in respect of ionic composition, pH and protein stabilization. If a labile virus is suspected, material should be transported on ice.

41.　B C E　　　　　　　　　　　Ref: 4,142

Norway and Sweden are rabies-free but Denmark is not. Areas isolated by water offer a prospect of being rabies-free and include the U.K., Japan and Australia but not Ceylon.

42.　A C D E　　　　　　　　　　Ref: 4,143-145

The incubation period ranges from 4 days to many years. usually 20 - 90 days. This patient is certainly still at risk. After infection there is no detectable immune response until symptoms develop. HDCSV is now the vaccine of choice and produces good antibody levels; however during the first week protection can be improved by giving HRIg.

43. **A B E**   Ref: 4,181

The tonsillar and intestinal forms which were formerly common in this country were due to the ingestion of tubercle bacilli, usually in milk, which is now only rarely a source of infection.

Infection is now usually by *inhalation* of droplet nuclei containing the organism, derived from infected sputum. The tuberculin response becomes positive some 4 to 6 weeks after infection. Patients (nearly always children) with primary tubercolosis seldom produce sputum and if bacteriological confirmation is required examination of gastric washings is necessary. Complications are rare but include pneumonia, pleurisy and bronchial compression by lymph nodes; more serious is haematogenous spread which may case miliary disease or later metastatic infection, especially in bones and joints.

44. **A B C E**   Ref: 2,504/178

Hand, foot and mouth disease is usually caused by the A16 virus but can also be due to the A5 or A10 viruses, or occasionally group B coxsackie viruses. Japanese B encephalitis is caused by one of the flavivirus group of arboviruses.

45. **A C E**   Ref: 4,176

The drug is selectively concentrated in keratin and only low concentrations are found in serum. There are no known resistant strains and resistance does not develop during treatment. It diminishes the action of anticoagulants but potentiates the action of alcohol.

46. **C**   Ref: 4,170-172

Acute pulmonary histoplasmosis is diagnosed by isolation of the organism (if possible) and by serology. Skin tests are of little value and can cause false positive serological tests.

In chronic disseminated histoplasmosis serology is often positive but usually in very low titre; culture of the oral ulcers or histology are more satisfactory. In North American blastomycosis, serology is negative in half the cases; culture is the most helpful procedure. The diagnosis of invasive aspergillosis is difficult; cultures are often negative and biopsy may be best. Serology is frequently negative even when sensitive techniques are used. There is no reliable skin test for cryptococcosis; diagnosis is by direct examination and culture and by serology.

47. **A C D**   Ref: 4,137,138

Amantidine is effective in both prophylaxis and in treatment (if started early enough), though pulmonary complications may not always be prevented. Intravenous idoxuridine is of no benefit in herpes encephalitis and carries a grave risk of bone marrow damage. Topical IDU is effective in superficial herpes eye infections. Intravenous vidarabine has reduced encephalitis mortality from 70% to 30% in one trial. Interferon is species-specific and the only benefits claimed so far have been from the use of human interferon.

48.   A C D   Ref: 4,148
The reservoir for dengue haemorrhagic fever is monkeys and that for Korean haemorrhagic fever is field rodents.

49.   A B C E   Ref: 5,189,190
Severe cases with septicaemia, circulatory collapse and massive pulmonary consolidation are now extremely rare. The organism, an intracellular parasite, was originally thought to be a virus but is now classified as a bacterum (Chlamydia); nevertheless viral techniques are required for its culture. Pneumonia is invariable but there may be little in the way of clinical signs.
Most patients are only diagnosed in retrospect, and usually recover without treatment. Tetracycline is effective but must be given early in the illness to be of any value.

50.   A B E   Ref: 5,190,191
Depression may occur in the chronic relapsing form. Conjunctivitis is seen in about 25% of patients with acute brucellosis.
Spondylitis and crippling arthritis are peculiar to *B.melitensis* infection.
The usual blood picture in acute abortus brucellosis is a lymphocytosis with a polymorph leucopenia. The organisms commonly lodge in reticulo-endothelial tissues, with involvement of the liver, spleen, bone marrow and lymph nodes.

51.   A B E   Ref: 5,192,193
The 'malignant pustule' is usually solitary and painless. The organisms can be readily demonstrated in smears from the eschar or from vesicular fluid; culture by guinea-pig inoculation is not without risk to laboratory staff. Vaccination of workers in the occupations mentioned eliminates the disease.

52.   B E   Ref: 5,193,194
Orf is a disease of *sheep and goats,* particularly young lambs.
In man the lesions occur on the hands and forearms of shepherds handling infected lambs; systemic symptoms may occur but are rare. Milkers' nodule is due to a similar, but distinct, virus which infects dairy cows. Treatment is symptomatic only.

53.   A B D   Ref: 5,194,195
Blood culture may be expected to be positive in the first week, but urine culture not until the third week. Penicillin is the drug of choice but has no effect if given after the first week. Domestic infection is from infected *dogs* (usually puppies).

54. **A B C D E**   Ref: 5,201
All the conditions mentioned can give false positive results with the non-specific or lipoidal tests for syphilis.

55. **A B D E**   Ref: 5,203,204,207
No generalized complications of N.S.U. have been described up to the present. Proctitis from which Chlamydia may be isolated is sometimes seen in homosexuals with a history of N.S.U. contact.

56. **B C D**   Ref: 5,204
Genital herpes is caused by *Herpesvirus hominis* Type II whereas ordinary lip herpes is caused by *H.hominis* Type I.
Penicillin and other treponemicidal drugs should NOT be given as they may confuse the diagnosis of coincidental syphilis.

57. **B C D E**   Ref: 5,208
The placental barrier is completely effective against nearly all bacterial and protozoal invaders (Toxoplasma is an exception) and in general only viruses can cross it.

58. **A C D**   Ref: 5,213,218
The activity of K-cells on antibody-coated cells is independent of complement. These cells play a part in the destruction of virus-infected cells, in renal homograft rejection, in auto-immune thyroiditis and probably in other autoimmune conditions.
They are morphologically similar to lymphocytes.

59. **B D E**   Ref: 5,227,230
The relation between the appropriate HLA typing and multiple sclerosis is not strong enough to be of diagnostic value. The finding of HLA-B27 is strong diagnostic evidence in favour of ankylosing spondylitis and might prove useful guide-lines in management at a very early stage. HBs - Ag positive hepatitis has no HLA association. In suspected myasthenia gravis, if the patient is negative for HLA-DR3 a thymoma is more probable and should be sought more diligently. A hypertensive woman who is positive for HLA-DR3 should not be treated with hydralazine since she has an increased risk of developing drug-induced SLE.

60. **A B C E**   Ref: 5,194.195
The initial (leptospiraemic) stage lasts for 4 - 7 days with influenza-like symptoms; these subside and 48 hours later the immune stage develops, with a secondary rise in temperature.
Blindness or blurred vision will clear up in a few days.
Penicillin is effective in the leptospiraemic stage only, and not in the immune stage.

61. **A D**   Ref: 5,198
The rash is macular at first but later becomes papular and finally papulo-squamous. The lesions spread to involve the face, the whole of the limbs and the palms and soles. Flexor surfaces are more involved than extensor.

62. **B D E**   Ref: 5,183
Person-to-person transmission is so uncommon that patients do not require isolation. In many outbreaks a common source has been identified, eg. contaminated air-conditioning water.
Peak incidence in Europe and N.America is in the late summer.
Retrospective studies have identified previous outbreaks as far back as 1947.

63. **B C**   Ref: 5,197,199,200
Late syphilis is usually defined as developing *two years* after the original infection. The tongue may be affected by diffuse gummatous infiltration. Treatment of late syphilis may destroy the spirochaetes but the changes already caused may lead to progressive damage eg. aneurysm formation. The term is equally applicable to congenital syphilis; an untreated affected child is considered to enter the 'late' stage on his or her second birthday.

64. **A B E**   Ref: 5,202
Bed rest in hospital is necessary, together with antibiotic therapy. Bacteriological confirmation should always be sought since some cases, clinically indistinguishable, are non-gonococcal in origin. Doubtful cases should be referred to a gynaecologist for laparascopy.

65. **B C D**   Ref: 1,37
The Sabin-Feldman dye test detects IgG antibody against toxoplasma. The Paul-Bunnell test is negative. Specific IgM antibody can also be detected using indirect immunofluorescence.
Isolation of the parasite is difficult but can be attempted by inoculating body fluids or tissue extracts into laboratory mice.
The passive haemagglutination test is useful as a screening test but does not provide *definitive* confirmation.

66. **A B D E**   Ref: 6,252
Patients with this syndrome are normovolaemic and therefore do not develop pulmonary oedema. Demeclocycline acts not on the pituitary gland but on the kidney, rendering it relatively insensitive to ADH. Fits and coma do not usually develop unless the plasma sodium falls below 110 mmol/1.

67. **A B**   Ref: 6,277
Therapy in an ill patient should be started at once, after blood has been taken for plasma urea, electrolytes and cortisol.
An abnormal short Synacthen test should be confirmed with a depot

Synacthen test. Adrenocortical antibodies are found in 80% of female patients with Addisons's disease but only in 10% of male patients.

68. **A B C** Ref: 6,274,275
Alcoholism may mimic Cushing's syndrome clinically. Metyrapone suppresses *cortisol* production and in Cushing's disease leads to a further increase in ACTH, which in turn causes an increase in urinary 17-oxogenic steroids. 20% of all patients with Cushing's disease have detectable enlargement of the pituitary fossa when first seen.

69. **B D** Ref: 6,275
Treatment is essential; there is a high morbidity from hypertension, heart disease, diabetes and osteoporosis in untreated cases. Metyrapone acts on the adrenal, blocking the synthesis of cortisol; it can therefore produce clinical remission in all spontaneous forms of the syndrome. The fall in plasma cortisol may be abrupt and profound and in the absence of a steroid supplement this could be dangerous. The treatment of choice for Cushing's disease is some form of pituitary ablation, either by surgery or by yttrium-90 implantation. Bilateral adrenalectomy is likely to be followed by Nelson's syndrome.

70. **A C D E** Ref: 6,232A (fig 2)
Angiotensin levels are increased in the erect posture.
Stress and anxiety activate the hypothalamic-pituitary-adrenal cortex system and increase the secretion of growth hormone and prolactin. Sodium depletion caused by diuretics activates the renin-angiotensin-alderosterone system.

71. **A B C E** Ref: 6,259,260
The duration of action of a dose of propranolol is about 6 hours. Rashes, and other side-effects such as arthralgia, jaundice and lymphadenopathy are usually transient and may respond to a short course of anti-histamines without withdrawal of the antithyroid drug; alternatively, another drug of the anti-thyroid group may be given.

72. **A D E** Ref: 6,260
Most authorities have given up trying to determine an exact dose and give an arbitrary dose (depending to some extent on the clinical size of the gland) with careful follow-up to determine the result. Up to 4 doses may be needed to achieve a cure.

73. **A D** Ref: 6,264.265
About 99.96% of T4 is protein bound. TBG concentration can be measured directly by radio-immuno-assay or immunoelectrophoresis.
The 'free thyroxine index', based on measurement of total T4 and of unoccupied protein-binding sites, is roughly proportional to the free T4 but is not a direct measurement of it. The T3 resin uptake test measures the

unoccupied binding sites and is quite unconnected with the plasma T3 level.

74.   C D E   Ref: 6,264,265
T4 is de-iodinated in the periphery to T3; the relative proportions arising by
this pathway and by release as T3 from the thyroid are not known. Reverse
T3 is similarly derived from T4. The rise in T3 toxicosis is due to increased
thyroid secretion rather than to increased tissue de-iodination. T3 levels
behave in much the same way as T4 levels in thyroid disturbances but
occasionally conversion of T4 to T3 is impaired, the 'low T3 syndrome'.

75.   AD   Ref: 7,306
The progestogen-only pill is less effective than the combined pill but there
are no serious adverse effects. The dose of progestogen is much *smaller* than
in the combined pill.

76.   A B D   Ref: 7,310
Synthetic androgens for oral use usually effect only partial replacement and
may cause cholestatic jaundice, possibly even hepatoma. High-dosage
androgen replacement may be complicated by polycythaemia and occasionally
by fluid retention. Prior treatment with androgens does not influence the
potential for stimulation with FSH when fertility is desired.

77.   A C E   Ref: 7,292
The effect of a rise in oestradiol secretion is to *increase* the pituitary
response to gonadotrophin-releasing hormone.

78.   A D   Ref: 7,295
Patients who have been amenorrhoeic for more than 10 years have
responded successfully to therapy. Bromocriptine may cause postural
hypotension. Its action is a direct one on the pituitary

79.   B D E   Ref: 7,288-290
The outlook with bilateral blockage is bad but not hopeless.
The success rate with extracorporeal fertilization is still extremely low even
in very skilled hands.

80.   A C D   Ref: 7,301

The effect of cyproterone acetate is to reduce libido and this may
occasionally be troublesome with high doses.
Clinical improvement will not be seen until after 6 months treatment at the
earliest.

81.   D E   Ref: 7,322
The karotype is 47, XXY. Spermatogenesis is always impaired.
Plasma testosterone levels are low to normal.

82.   **B D E**   Ref: 8,359.361
Routine determination of the individual lipo-proteins is time-consuming and
expensive and the measurement of plasma cholesterol and triglyceride
levels after a 12 - 24 hour over-night fast is usually sufficient. Isolated
elevation of plasma triglyceride indicates a rise in VLDL.

83.   **A C D E**   Ref: 8,360.361
Pancreatitis occurs in patients with high triglyceride levels (chylomicronaemia)
and control of the latter will reduce the frequency of attacks of pancreatitis.

84.   **B**   Ref: 8,344,345
Hyperventilation is a feature of both conditions. The drugs predisposing to
lactic acidosis are the biguanide group, especially phenformin. The blood
pressure may be low in both conditions. A cold clammy skin would suggest
hypoglycaemic coma; in both the acidotic states the skin is usually warm.

85.   **B C E**   Ref: 8,338
Patients with mild sensory neuropathy have no symptoms; an absent ankle
jerk may be the only clinical abnormality.

86.   **B C D E**   Ref: 8,342
Non-selective β-blockers can mask warning symptoms of hypoglycaemia in
patients on insulin. Aldomet, bethanidine and guanethiudine may all
precipitate postural hypotension due to autonomic neuropathy. In diabetes
with autonomic neuropathy several factors, including anaesthesia, respiratory
depressant drugs and respiratory infections, are thought to be responsible
for causing cardio-respiratory arrest. Thiazide diuretics may worsen blood-
sugar control in non-insulin dependent diabetes.

87.   **A B**   Ref: 8,332
Haemolytic anaemia etc. will cause falsely low values of GHb; some
haemoglobinopathies cause falsely high values. There is no advantage of
methods measuring special fractions or precursors over the measurement of
total GHb.

88.   **C D**   Ref: 8,327,328
A two-hour blood glucose of less than 6 mmol/l excludes diabetes.
In the absence of diabetic symptoms at least two abnormal values are
required to establish the diagnosis of diabetes. Impaired glucose tolerance
in pregnancy must be taken very seriously and treated as diabetes.

89.   **A C D E**   Ref: 8,329
Retinopathy, nephropathy and arterial disease are all less common in
'flushers' than in 'non-flushers'.

90.   **B D E**   Ref: 8,351
Brain tissue can utilize ketone bodies but the development of significant
ketosis requires several hours in man. If the hypoglycaemia is due to excess

insulin this will inhibit ketogenesis. Patients with long-standing diabetes are likely to develop autonomic neuropathy and therefore to have less severe adrenergic symptoms. In patients with insulinomas the blood sugar level usually drops slowly and this produces neurological rather than adrenergic symptoms.

91.   **A D E**   **Ref: 8,353.354**
In the presence of low blood glucose insulin secretion is largely suppressed. Hence the finding of low fasting glucose and high fasting insulin levels is diagnostic of insulinoma or self-medication with insulin or a sulphonylurea drug. Only about 10% are malignant.

92.   **A C**   **Ref: 9,376**
The specified errors of technique would cause on the one hand the loss of plasma ultrafiltrate (hence a rise in all proteins and protein bound substances) and on the other the release of muscle constituents including lactate, pyruvate, lactate dehydrogenase and creatine kinase. Glucose and sodium are not affected. Serum acid phosphatase would be elevated by haemolysis and by delay in separating the serum.

93.   **A B D**   **Ref: 9,379.390**
Recent fracture, Paget's disease and a high alcohol intake will all raise the alkaline phosphatase, which in any case tends to rise in normal elderly subjects. Exposure of the serum to light, especially UV, will *decrease* the level of *bilirubin.*

94.   **B E**   **Ref: 9,407,408**
Chronic lead poisoning causes constipation with abdominal cramps. The lead in the blood is mostly in the red cells, therefore whole blood samples are used for analysis. Sodium-calcium edetate is given intravenously.

95.   **A D**   **Ref: 9,408,409**
Mercury vapour inhalation usually produces an acute respiratory reaction with cough, wheezing and dyspnoea which resolves within 24 hours or so. Following ingestion of mercuric chloride, if the patient survives the initial diarrhoea and shock, there is a serious risk of acute renal failure. Gastric aspiration should be avoided if possible because of the friability of the stomach wall.

96.   **A D**   **Ref: 9,404.405**
The possible ingested dose amounts to 750mg; anything over 500 mg warrants intensive care. Gastric lavage is worthwhile up to 24 hours after ingestion. Most disturbance of the ECG can be corrected by attention to oxygenation and correction of acidosis; over-zealous administration of anti-arrythmic agents before they are needed may be harmful....A serious cardiac hazard, that of arrest, arises from the conduction defects caused by the drug, and apart from tachyarrhythmais, intraventricular conduction block, as

shown by widened QRS complexes, should be sought and monitoring continued until the QRS duration as been reduced to 0.1 sec. for at least 12 hours.

97. **A B C D E**   Ref: 9,413,414

Both chlorinated (B,C) and fluorinated (D,E) hydrocarbons sensitize the heart to circulating catecholamines. Death from inhalation of petrol vapour is rare but its aromatic fractions may have a similar effect on the heart and so cause ventricular fibrillation.

98. **B C E**   Ref: 9,U109

Water hemlock poisoning causes profuse vomiting, hyperventilation and muscle spasms. *A. phalloides* also causes vomiting, diarrhoea and a variety of biochemical disturbances including hepatic and renal failure.

99. **A B C**   Ref: 9,389-391

In Cushing's syndrome excessive corticosteroid secretion is responsible, and in Klinefelter's syndrome low androgen levels.
The effect of calcitonin and of fluoride is to reduce bone breakdown.

100. **B C D**   Ref: 9: 392,393

The serum 25-OHC is almost invariably lowered and often undetectable. 1000 - 2000 I.U. daily of Vitamin D is sufficient to cure nutritional osteomalacia but if malabsorption is the cause daily doses of the order of 5000 I.U. or more are needed.

101. **C D**   Ref: 9,394

Osteopetrosis with recessive inheritance is a severe condition and manifests itself within the first year of life; the bones are fragile and fractures are usual. Compression of the marrow cavity leads to anaemia and thrombocytopenia. The basic defect is thought to be a deficiency of *osteoclasts* and success has been claimed for bone marrow transplantation providing osteo-clast precursors.

102. **A B**   Ref: 9,394

The bone lesions are usually asymmetrical and the bones most often affected are the femur and tibia. The skin may show *increased* pigmentation ('cafe-au-lait spots').

103. **A D E**   Ref: 9,381,382

Protein malnutrition and cirrhosis may both cause low plasma albumin and consequent oedema. Paralytic ileus causes loss of tissue fluid (containing sodium) into the bowel lumen and diabetes causes an osmotic diuresis with loss of sodium in the urine. Filariasis causes lymphatic obstruction and hence oedema.

104. **B C**   Ref: 9,383
There are no warning symptoms or signs; unless a serum potassium estimation is deliberately requested the first indication of hyperkalaemia may be a cardiac arrest. The quickest protective procedure is the intravenous injection of calcium salts eg. gluconate. The expected acid-base disturbance would be acidosis; the desired change would be a shift towards the alkaline side, which causes the potassium to move from extracellular fluid into cells.

105. **A B D E**   Ref: 9,383,384
Intestinal obstruction produces potassium depletion through prolonged vomiting. Amiloride is a potassium-sparing diuretic.
Malignant hypertension may cause secondary hyper-aldosteronism and carcinoma of the bronchus may cause ectopic ACTH secretion with consequent over-secretion of cortisol.

106. **A C D**   Ref: 9,397.398
In patients taking chlorpropamide, phenylbutazone will cause enzyme inhibition with potentiation of the drug and hypoglycaemia.
Chloroquine and oestrogens may precipitate porphyria but do not interfere with diabetes. In patients on insulin, propranolol prevents hepatic glycogenolysis and blocks adrenergic responses, thus prolonging hypoglycaemia and masking its clinical manifestations. Chloramphenicol inhibits enzymatic destruction of tolbutamide and so can cause hypoglycaemia.

107. **A D E**   Ref: 9,415,417
Heparin should not be used as venom causes capillary wall damage. Morphine is contraindicated and diazepam is effective as a sedative. Freezing and incision cause unnecessary damage and are ineffective; firm pressure over the bite, and immobilization if it is on a limb, is the best procedure.

108. **A D**   Ref: 10,457,458
Nerve and tendon compression require priority treatment because of the need to forestall paralysis, sensory loss and tendon rupture. Upper limb surgery should be carried out first so that crutches can be used to reduce weight-bearing on a recently-repaired lower limb joint. Arthrodesis of the wrist can produce a stable painless joint with excellent function. The ruptured tendon (usually that of the little finger) should be sutured to the adjacent intact ones.

109. **B D E**   Ref: 10,446
Radiology is of little help in early diagnosis. Surgical drainage should only be considered if there has been a delay in diagnosis or antibiotic therapy has failed to produce an improvement.

110. **B E** Ref: 10,446

The characteristic rash is erythema marginatum; erythema nodosum would be more suggestive of sarcoidosis. The ESR is always raised in the absence of cardiac failure. Pericarditis is not diagnostic; it can also occur in systemic juvenile chronic arthritis, SLE and viral infections. Subcutaneous nodules over the elbows and knees may be seen in rheumatic fever.

111. **B C D** Ref: 10,447,448

Only about 10% of children have an illness resembling adult rheumatoid arthritis, and these are the only group in which rheumatoid factor is found. There is a strong association between the presence of ANA in the serum and chronic iridocyclitis.

112. **C E** Ref: 10,449

Prolonged bed rest should be discouraged. Arthritic children often excel in water sports and swimming should be actively encouraged. Gold is effective in juvenile arthritis but carries the same risks as in adults.

113. **A B C D E** Ref: 10,450

The rash may be urticarial or ecchymotic and tends to appear on the buttocks with continuation on to the extensor surfaces of the legs.
The ESR may be normal initially, even in the presence of a raised level of IgA. Haemorrhage into the gut wall causes abdominal pain and occasionally melaena.

114. **B C D** Ref: 10,431

Nodules may also develop in tendon sheaths, lung, pleura, myocardium, pericardium and sclera. They occur in about 20% of cases.

115. **A B C D E** Ref: 10,433

Splenomegaly, neutropenia, thrombocytopenia and anaemia are the classic findings in Felty's syndrome. The remaining features are less common but well recognized. These patients are at risk of recurrent and severe infections.

116. **A C** Ref: 10,463,464

The dramatic effect of phenylbutazone in ankylosing spondylitis is due to its powerful anti-inflammatory activity and not to any specific curative effect. There is little evidence of synergism between drugs of different groups. Modified salicylic acid preparations eg. salsalate and trilisate, are longer-acting and can be given twice daily.

117. **A C D E** Ref: 10,465,466

Penicillamine is effective in rheumatoid arthritis, palindromic rheumatism and some types of juvenile chronic arthritis, but not in juvenile ankylosing spondylitis, psoriatic arthropathy or any other inflammatory arthritis. A rare but dangerous toxic effect is pancytopenia and if serial white cell or platelet counts show a consistent downward trend the drug must be withdrawn permanently.

On the other hand the early maculo-papular rash is not serious, disappearing quickly when the drug is withdrawn and seldom recurring when it is re-introduced.

118. A C   Ref: 10,468

Azathroprine may be particularly useful for patients not responding to penicillamine, since they may also fail to respond to gold. It does not cause infertility. It is broken down by xanthine oxidase, which is inhibited by allopurinol; hence patients on allopurinol should be given a much *smaller* dose of azathroprine, about one-quarter of the normal.

119. B C D E   Ref: 10,468

Chloroquine does not retard the progression of radiological change.

The dose-related retinopathy it causes is difficult to distinguish from the retinopathy of advancing age, hence the need for caution in older patients.

120. A D E   Ref: 10,437

Only about 1% of all subjects with HLA-B27 develop ankylosing spondylitis; of those *with the disease* 96% have HLA-B27. The pain is worst on waking and is made better by exercise. Pain from involvement of the costo-vertebral joints resembles that of pleurisy, but is usually bilateral and comes and goes in episodes.

121. C D E   Ref: 10,440

In both ulcerative colitis and Crohn's disease the incidence of arthritis is equal in men and women. The commonest presentation is as a mono-arthritis of the knee. Intra-articular injection of steroids may be valuable if drug administration is limited by the bowel disease.

122. C   Ref: 10,454

Arthrodesis is relatively free from long-term complications and this may tilt the balance in favour of its selection in younger patients. In the wrist, ankle and metacarpophalangeal joint of the thumb it causes little disability. In the hip a unilateral arthrodesis may be possible but replacement gives excellent short-term results and is virtually the only possible procedure if both hips are involved.

123. A C   Ref:10,454

Penicillin improves the symptoms of Whipple's disease within days. Venesection, although beneficial as regards other manifestations of haemochromatosis, seems to have no effect on the arthropathy. The joint manifestations of hypothyroidism, including knee effusions, respond rapidly and completely to replacement therapy. The appropriate therapy for familial Mediterranean fever is prophylaxis with colchicine. No treatment is available for Fabry's disease, a rare condition due to accumulation in the tissues of glycolipids.

125
~~124.~~ **A E** Ref: 11,500-502
In the presence of renal involvement, it is important to identify membranous or diffuse proliferative glomerulonephritis, since the patients with the latter should be given immuno-suppressive drugs in addition to steroids. The ANA test is suitable for screening only; the most specific test is that for antibodies to double-stranded DNA. Although SLE is a classic example of immune-complex disease, serial estimation of complex levels is not a good guide to management. The EEG is often abnormal in the absence of overt cerebral disease.

124
~~125.~~ **A C E** Ref: 11,504,505
Cerebral disease and renal disease are uncommon. DNA-binding antibodies are usually absent, but there is a high titre of antibodies to ribonucleoprotein.

126. **A D E** Ref:11,506
There is a normochromic anaemia and a raised ESR but usually no leucytosis. There is *tenderness* of proximal muscles but not weakness. The illness may be a manifestation of occult malignancy, early rheumatoid arthritis or bacterial endocarditis.

127. **C D** Ref: 11,U120
Conjunctivitis and tenosynovitis are seen in both conditions.
Demonstration of gonococci is often difficult in gonococcal arthritis; conversely, gonococci may be found incidentally in patients with Reiter's syndrome.

128. **A E** Ref: 11,513
Hydroxyproline excretion is an index of collagen breakdown, and since in Paget's disease there is increased osteolysis (involving breakdown of bone collagen) the hydroxyproline excretion is increased. Hypercalcaemia only occurs during immobilization and is not a characteristic feature. The calcium-regulating hormone levels are normal.

129. **B C D** Ref:11,508-511
Evacuation of a haematoma is rarely necessary. Myositis ossificans is a rare and unpredictable sequel. Non-steroidal anti-inflammatory drugs probably have their greatest effect in the first few days. Physiotherapy is of no value in the painful phase of a 'frozen shoulder' and often exacerbates symptoms.

130. **B D E** Ref: 11,488
Bone density appears unchanged until 50% of the mineral has disappeared. The appearances are *normal* in 25% of patients with early ankylosing spondylitis.

131.   A C D E   Ref:11,488

Compression of a single nerve root is the characteristic finding in disc prolapse; involvement of *more than one* root would cast doubt on the diagnosis. Unremitting pain which is worse at night suggests tumour, infection or metabolic disease.

132.   B C E   Ref: 11,493

The proximal interphalangeal joints may also be affected. In the cervical spine osteophytes may encroach on the intervertebral foramina and compress the nerve-roots, and oblique views are required to demonstrate this. In the metatarsophalangeal joint of the big toe osteoarthritis may be accompanied by pseudo-cyst formation and this may be confused with the erosions of gout. In the knee, narrowing of the *medial* compartment is the commonest change.

133.   C   Ref: 11,494

Swimming is very valuable in promoting muscle strength and tone. The walking-stick should be in the hand *opposite* the painful joint. Walking frames are only used in the early stages after hip or knee surgery. Anti-inflammatory drugs are valuable as well as analgesics.

134.   A D E   Ref: 11,515

Taking 2 standard deviations above the mean as the upper limit of normal, the figure for males is 0.42 mmol/1 (7mg/100ml). The non-specific automated methods give results which are slightly higher than those given by the uricase method; in doubtful cases the latter must be used.

135.   A C E   Ref: 11,517

No alteration in sensible diet and drinking habits is necessary, but the weight should be reduced to normal if it is raised.

Allopurinol and uricosuric drugs should be withheld for several weeks after an acute attacks as they may trigger further attacks.

Anti-gout prophylactic therapy for the first 3 months is based on the same reasoning.

136.   B C E   Ref: 11,471,472

Rheumatoid factor antibody specificity is directed against sites on the Fc portion of the heavy chain of IgG. The standard laboratory tests detect only the IgM antiglobulins and these are what is meant when the term 'rheumatoid factor' is used without qualification. Immune complex formation and complement activation in synovial fluid have been observed, but it is thought that this is not the sole explanation for the inflammation within the joint.

137.   A B D   Ref: 11,474

IgG and IgA rheumatoid factors may be found in seronegative rheumatoid arthritis and in other sero-negative arthritides such as ankylosing spondylitis, psoriatic arthritis and juvenile chronic arthritis. About 5% of normal individuals, particularly those in older age groups, have a positive rheumatoid factor test.

138. **A B D** Ref: 12,538,539

In upper gastro-intestinal bleeding the source can be identified by endoscopy in 90% of patients; the corresponding figure for barium meal examination is 70%. Some 15% of gastric ulcers which by X-ray appear benign are in fact malignant. In patients with symptoms of peptic ulceration endoscopy reveals lesions in about 30% of those in whom the barium meal is normal. Hypoxaemia in patients with obstructive airways disease may precipitate cardiac arrhythmias. Perforation of the oesophagus usually requires surgery, although conservative management is possible.

139. **A B D** Ref: 12,552

In addition to eosinophilia of the peripheral blood there is dense eosinophilic infiltration of the mucosa and the muscularis mucosae of the stomach and to a lesser extent of the small intestine, where there may also be villous shortening and crypt hyperplasia. There is an associated iron deficiency anaemia.

140. **(All false).** Ref; 12,557

Appendicitis may be present with a normal leucocyte count.

Amylase may be normal with overwhelming pancreatitis and with pancreatitis caused by trauma. Gas is not seen in about 25% of cases of perforation. Only about 10% of gall-stones are radio opaque. In obstruction the obstructed loop is sometimes entirely filled with fluid and no levels are then seen.

141. **A B** Ref: 12,531,532

Laxatives will help to avoid faecal impaction with masses of barium sulphate. A patient with a phaeochromocytoma should not be given glucagon, which is used to promote relaxation of the gut. Single contrast barium meal examination may be expected to miss some 20% of abnormalities. Double contrast technique is valuable in examination of the duodenum as well as the stomach. The aim of pre-medication is to produce relaxation of the bowel, hence anti-cholinergic drugs are used.

142. **A C D** Ref: 12,526,527

Biopsy from a 'leather-bottle' stomach may yield fibrous tissue only. The changes of repair at the edge of a healing peptic ulcer need to be distinguished from the appearances or carcinoma.

'Gastritis' is a histopathological diagnosis which does not necessarily correlate with a clinical diagnosis of non-ulcer dyspepsia.

143. **B C D E** Ref: 12,520

Belching is nearly always the regurgitation of air that has been swallowed, but in two situations the gas may be generated inside the stomach: (1) after taking large doses of sodium bicarbonate (2) very rarely with long-standing pyloric stenosis fermentation of food may take place within the stomach.

144.　C E　　　　　　　　　　　Ref: 13,575,576

There is no convincing evidence that psychological stress, steroid drugs or analgesics cause duodenal ulceration. Duodenal ulcer is uncommon in pregnancy. Smoking causes a small but definite increase in the incidence of duodenal ulcers.

145.　A B D　　　　　　　　　　Ref: 13,578

Endoscopy is needed to confirm the presence of an active ulcer. A raised gastrin level is consistent with the diagnosis of Zollinger-Ellison syndrome due to a gastrin-secreting pancreatic adenoma.

Increased doses of cimetidine are worth trying. A poor response to medical treatment does not mean that surgery will be equally unsatisfactory.

146.　B C E　　　　　　　　　　Ref: 13,579

The operation of choice for uncomplicated duodenal ulcer is proximal gastric vagotomy. Barium meal examination is made difficult by the distortion due to surgery; endoscopy is required. The patient's symptoms are unreliable since some patients develop ulcer symptoms with normal endoscopy and others may have pain-free recurrences which may present with haemorrhage.

147.　C　　　　　　　　　　　　Ref: 13,597,599

There is evidence of substantial blood loss and the most urgent need is for resuscitation. The absence of anaemia simply means that there has not been time for haemodilution to develop. There is no evidence that cimetidine is beneficial in this situation.

Surgery, if indicated, should be performed within 24 hours of admission if possible.

148.　A　　　　　　　　　　　　Ref: 13,601,602

The bleeding is usually bright red or plum-coloured but may present as melaena. The diverticulum is situated in the ileum and so is not visible with the colonoscope.

149.　A B C E　　　　　　　　　Ref: 13,604

Dermatitis herpetiformis is commonly accompanied by gluten enteropathy, in which malabsorption of vitamin K may cause bleeding. Pseudoxanthoma elasticum is associated with characteristic retinal lesions and with a tendency towards gastrointestinal bleeding. Acanthosis nigricans should always prompt a search for occult carcinoma; the tumour may be in the colon and may be the source of the bleeding. Psoriasis is not associated with any abnormality of the alimentary tract. In neurofibromatosis there may be associated intestinal fibromata which may be the source of occult blood loss.

150. **A D E**   Ref: 13,585
The result of digestion of polysaccharides by amylase is a mixture of maltose, maltriose and α-limit dextrins; further break-down of these, and of sucrose and lactose, does not occur in the lumen but is carried out by brush border enzymes. After breakdown of fat by pancreatic lipase into fatty acids and monoglycerides, bile salts act to make these water-soluble but are not themselves absorbed at this point; they are passed down to the terminal ileum and are absorbed there. After entry into mucosal cells the fatty acids and monoglycerides are resynthesized into triglyceride, coated with phospholipid and protein and passed out via the lacteals into the bloodstream as chylomicrons.

151. **A B C E**   Ref: 13,592
Rice, maize and soya can be used as substitutes; all the others contain gluten.

152. **A B D E**   Ref: 13,593,595
In tropical sprue tetracycline (with folic acid) is the treatment of choice. For Whipple's disease various antibiotics have been used, eg. penicillin and streptomycin for 2 weeks initially followed by tetracycline for 1 year. The treatment for intestinal lymphangiectasia is replacement of dietary fat by medium chain triglyceride.

153. **A B D E**   Ref: 13,571
All except lead poisoning are associated with carcinoma.

154. **B**   Ref: 14,636,637
The pain is felt in the upper abdomen. Diarrhoea may occur as a result of malabsorption. In younger patients fibro-muscular hyperplasia may be a cause. No clinical test exists to confirm the diagnosis of ischaemia.

155. **A D E**   Ref: 14,629
Estimation of CEA is unrealiable and has no place in the diagnosis of carcinoma of the colon. The surgical treatment of choice is wide resection of the affected colon with end-to-end anastomosis.

156. **A B C**   Ref: 14,621
The management of the disease in children is similar to that of adults. If long courses of treatment are necessary an alternate-day regime is advisable. Pregnancy does not affect the disease, though there may be a tendency to relapse in the puerperium.

157. **A D**   Ref: 14,646
The incidence of volvulus shows a negative correlation with diverticular disease. There is usually cramping abdominal pain and a plain X-ray shows the dilated colonic loop. If there is no evidence of peritonitis, decompression and detorsion should be attempted by proctoscopy.

158. A C   Ref:15,701
The mortality of common bile duct exploration in patients over 60 is 5-10%.
Endoscopic sphincterotomy causes immediate complications in about 7%
of patients and about half of these require surgical intervention. The chief
indication is removal of duct stones in patients who have had cholecystectomy
but it is also being used in patients with cholangitis or pancreatitis who still
have a gall-bladder.

159. A C D   Ref: 15,702
Many patients (70-100%) have Sjogren's syndrome, in which there is
diminished lacrimal and salivary secretion; pancreatic hypo-secretion also
occurs. Hyposecretion of the bronchial and sweat glands is found in
mucoviscidosis.

160. C D   Ref: 15,703,704
ERCP may be valuable in ruling out common bile duct pathology.
High levels of serum cholesterol are usual and reflect biliary obstruction
combined with good liver cell function. Aspartate transaminase levels show
only slight or moderate elevation and this helps to distinguish PBC from
other forms of chronic hepatitis.

161. A B D E   Ref: 15,709,710
In Felty's syndrome there is lymphocytic infiltration and regenerative
hyperplasia which sometimes progresses to macronodular cirrhosis. In
Still's disease hepatosplenomegaly is common, with abnormal liver function
tests and sometimes overt jaundice. Liver pathology is common in cystic
fibrosis but in childhood it is usually symptomless; in patients surviving to
adolescence cirrhosis may develop, sometimes with bleeding from varices.
Hepatomegaly, often with splenomegaly, is common in both primary and
secondary amyloidosis.

162. A B D E   Ref: 15,705
The mortality from cirrhosis among doctors is nearly twice that among
judges and lawyers. Taxation on alcohol in Scandina was shown to have
little influence on the incidence of alcoholic liver disease. The safe upper
intake limit is thought to be about 60 g of alcohol a day for men and 20 - 30 g
for women; this difference between the sexes is unexplained.

163. A B E   Ref: 15,690
A low serum calcium indicates extensive fat necrosis. Multiple fluid levels
on X-ray are very unusual and suggest intestinal obstruction. Hyperlipaemia
is usually a non-specific response to pancreatitis per se; familial
hyperlipaemia is a known cause of pancreatitis but an uncommon one.

164. B E   Ref: 15,692
Acute diabetes during an attack is usually self-limiting. Ketosis is
uncommon and there is a danger of irreversible insulin-induced

hypoglycaemia, so undertreatment is safer than overtreatment. The serum amylase may be normal. Fat necrosis occasionally involves subcutaneous fat.

165. **D E**   Ref: 15,696,697
Some 10 - 30% of gall-stones are radio-opaque. CT scanning has proved disappointing as a method of detection. Failure to visualize the gall bladder on oral cholecytography may be due to poor absorption and in 10% of such cases the result of a repeat examination is normal.

166. **B D**   Ref: 16,741,742
Ibuprofen may cause dose-independent hepatic necrosis.
Amitriptyline is a tricyclic antidepressant; all drugs of this group may cause cholestatic jaundice. Iproniazid, a mono-amine oxidase inhibitor, may cause hepatic necrosis. Tetracycline, if given in large doses (more than 2 g by mouth daily) may cause central and mid-zonal hepatic necrosis.

167. **A B C D**   Ref: 16,743
Results of monitoring during treatment may be difficult to assess if the state of the patient's hepatic function before treatment is not known. Liver function tests in the first three months may give early warning of a reaction to isoniazid.
Rifampicin is a potent enzme-inducing agent and a rise in γ-glutamyl-transferase is not evidence per se of liver damage.

168. **B D E**   Ref: 16,756
The usual presentation is acute with fever and pain in the right hypochondrium. The quickest test is the latex agglutination test (10 minutes).

169. **A B D**   Ref: 16,735,736
Amiloride, a potassium-sparing diuretic, is very effective, especially in combination with a potassium-losing diuretic such as frusemide. In a patient with severe portal hypertension, well-preserved liver function and intractable ascites, a portacaval shunt may be the best means of providing relief.

170. **B C**   Ref: 16,723,724
Faecal shedding of HAV is short-lived and may be complete by the time the patient is seen. The best test is the demonstration of hepatitis-A-specific IgM. There are no specific tests for non-A, non-B hapatitis; the diagnosis is made by exclusion of HAV, HBV, cytomegalovirus and Epstein-Barr virus. HBcAg (the core component) is useful in diagnosis.

171. **B C D**   Ref: 16,725
Non-A non-B hepatitis is a common complication of blood transfusion. There is some evidence that human normal immunoglobulin may be protective but its role is still unclear.

172. **B D E** Ref: 16,737-739
Recovery may be complete, with restoration of normal liver structure. The bleeding tendency is due to a multitude of causes, including inadequate synthesis of coagulation factors, lack of vitamin K and reduced platelets; fibrinolysis may occur but it is uncommon and certainly not the main cause. Hyperventilation may occur in the early stages but there may also be sudden and unexpected respiratory arrest.

173. **C** Ref: 16,726,727
Vascular spiders and splenomegaly are not seen., The serum IgG is normal, an important distinction from chronic active hepatitis.
Cirrhosis does not develop.

174. **C E** Ref: 16,728
Bed rest is unnecessary unless symptoms are severe; no dietary restrictions are needed except avoidance of alcohol. Corticosteroids in theory might favour viral replication and the later development of carcinoma; nevertheless in severe cases they may be beneficial. In asymptomatic cases careful observation for some months is desirable before starting steroids, and they are particularly unsuitable for the very young, the very old and those with diabetes.

175. **A D** Ref: 16,718,719
A platelet count over $80 \times 10^9/1$ would be acceptable as would a haemoglobin over 10g/1. Biopsy is an established method of confirming the diagnosis of hepatic cancer and the only tumour involving added risk is haemangioma.

176. **A B** Ref: 16,754,755
The last three are benign tumours. Removal of focal nodular hyperplastic tissue is seldom necessary but perfectly feasible if it is causing symptoms.

177. **A C** Ref: 16,731,732
Storage of blood reduces the concentration of clotting factors and the number of platelets, and increases the concentration of ammonia and potassium. Bleeding is from a non-variceal site in some 50% of patients with portal hypertension due to cirrhosis, and endoscopic confirmation of variceal bleeding is essential. Vasopressin may cause coronary artery constriction.
Endoscopic injection is unreliable and trans-hepatic injection or embolization is more effective.

178. **D** Ref: 17,791,792
Bradycardia is an indication of effective β-blockade and a heart-rate of 40 per minute with no accompanying symptoms should be disregarded. Partial agonist activity will not prevent heart failure. Propranolol is not cardioselective.

Atenolol is a hydrophilic drug and so is less likely than lipophilic drugs to penetrate the CNS and cause nightmares and depression.

179. **A D**   Ref: 17,791,792

Nadolol and sotalol are hydrophilic, are not broken down in the liver and have long plasma half-lives (20 and 16 hours respectively). The remaining drugs are lipophilic and have plasma half-lives of 2 - 3 hours.

180. **A B D**   Ref: 17,793

AV re-entrant tachycardia and hypertrophic cardiomyopathy are both indications for the use of verapamil. If given I.V. in the presence of β-blockade severe bradycardia or hypotension may develop, sometimes with a fatal result. In patients with digitalis toxicity there is a risk of heart block; if verapamil must be given in this situation, a pacing wire must be inserted first.

181. **A C D**   Ref: 17,795

Cholestyramine and kaolin-pectin mixtures bind digitalia drugs in the gut lumen, impair intestinal absorption of the drug and reduce the therapeutic effect. Amphotericin B may cause hypokalaemia and hence digitalis toxicity. Nifedipine and quinidine impair renal excretion of digitalis and hence may cause toxicity.

182. **A C D E**   Ref: 17,794,796

Digoxin is excreted unchanged by the kidney and undergoes little or no metabolism in the intestine or liver. The remaining drugs undergo oxidation or conjugation in the liver and 'first-pass metabolism' accounts for a substantial proportion of their total removal.

183. **B C D**   Ref: 17,786,787

Central chest pain which is worse on deep inspiration and relieved by sitting forward suggests acute pericarditis. Left inframammary pain suggests effort syndrome. A heavy meal and exposure to cold are well-known factors which precipitate or favour ischaemic cardiac pain.

184. **A B**   Ref: 17,775,776,778

Measuremenmt of ventricular wall thickness is best done with M-mode. Pericardial constriction and left atrial myxoma can be detected equally well by either technieque.

185. **B C D**   Ref: 17,770,771

There may be considerable hypertrophy of the left ventricle in aortic stenosis without producing diagnostic change in the cardiac outline. Bronchial arterial enhancement only occurs as a result of pulmonary arterial oligaemia, eg. in pulmonary atresia.

186. A D E   Ref: 17,779
Injection of labelled microspheres is suitable for measurement of a right-to-left shunt. Myocardial infarction is assessed from the uptake of technetium-99m pyrophosphate.

187. A B C D E   Ref: 17,803
Patients with the sick-sinus syndrome may be abnormally sensitive to digoxin, β-blockers and verapamil. DC shock may suppress sinus node function.

188. A D E   Ref: 17,804
The arrhythmia is intermittent, 5 to 30 beats at a time, then reverting to sinus rhythm. The prognosis is not made worse and treatment is unnecessary unless the rate is very fast or cardiac performance deteriorates.

189. A B D   Ref: 17,804
The rhythm may be slightly irregular. If SVT is accompanied by bundle-branch block the ECG may resemble that of VT. Short bursts of VT do not necessarily presage more dangerous arrhythmias.

190   B D E   Ref: 17,764
An rSR pattern over the right precordium is characteristic of right bundle branch block. The axis in LBBB usually lies between 0° and -45°. Deep S waves in lead 1 and the left precordial leads are suggestive of RBBB. Abnormal repolarization leads to ST depression and T wave inversion over the left ventricle.

191. All false   Ref: 18,846,847
In general the patient should keep warm; reflex heating may be of benefit in frost-bite and in acute secondary Raynaud's disease.

192. A C D E   Ref: 18,841
In venography the contrast material is injected into a foot vein; this is often painful and the procedure may initiate thrombosis or may dislodge an existing thrombus. The labelled fibrinogen test depends on uptake of fibrinogen by the developing thrombus and therefore requires a day or more before a positive result can be detected with certainty.

193. A B C   Ref: 18,814
The dangerous rhythms are those which are likely to lead to ventricular arrest.

194. A B E   Ref: 18,836,837
Renewal of a driving licence for HGV's will almost certainly not be granted. There is no bar to sexual activity.

195. **A B E**   Ref: 18,817
The age of onset ranges from 6 to 15 years with a peak at 8 years.
There is no sex difference in incidence. RF is commoner in children of
parents with RHD than in non-related adopted children or children of non-
affected parents and is 3 times commoner in monozygotic than in dizygotic
twins. The incidence in developed countries is 0.5 - 1 per 1000 while in
developing countries it ranges from 7 to 33 per 1000.

196. **A B C**   Ref: 18,818
Aortic stenosis does not occur with the initial attack; basal ejection systolic
murmurs are functional. The tachycardia is usually *greater* than expected
for a given degree of fever.

197. **A B D E**   Ref: 18,830-832
Aortic stenosis causes concentric hypertrophy of the ventricle with a small
cavity, hence there is at first no enlargement of the cardiac outline.

198. **A B E**   Ref: 18,821
The normal valve area is 4 - 6 cm²; there are no symptoms until it has been
reduced to 2.5 cm². Reduction to 1 cm² represents a critical state. Some
20% of patients with systemic embolism are in regular rhythm. Pain similar
in character and distribution to that of angina pectoris is found in some 15%
of patients with mitral stenosis and normal coronary arteries; the cause is
uncertain but the pain is usually relieved by valvotomy.
The apex beat is not displaced unless there is associated mitral regurgitation,
aortic valve disease or systemic hypertension.

199. **A B C E**   Ref: 18,826
Cardiac defects are not recognized consequences of Klinefelter's syndrome.

200. **A B C E**   Ref: 18,813
If a fixed-rate pacemaker is implanted when spontaneous cardiac activity is
still present (conducted beats, extrasystoles) the pacemaker impulse may
fall in the period of spontaneous depolarization and induce ventricular
fibrillation. In temporary block due to cardiac infarction a demand
pacemaker is essential for this very reason, since the block will probably
recover.

201. **C**   Ref: 19,880
All the findings except rapid development of heart failure are characteristic
of *chronic* aortic regurgitation. Aortic valve destruction in infective
endocarditis is rapid and gives no time for the development of the chronic
changes.

202. **A D E**   Ref: 19,884
Cyanosis due to tricuspid atresia or to pulmonary atresia with intact
ventricular septum is usually obvious within the first month of life.

203.   A B D   Ref: 19,888
A pulmonary systolic thrill is uncommon and should suggest the presence of associated pulmonary stenosis. The prognosis is good during childhood and cardiac failure does not usually develop until adult life.

204.   A E   Ref: 19,858
There is no evidence of a diminishing response to long-term digoxin. Rapid loading confers no advantage; in particular, intravenous digoxin causes potentially dangerous arterial vasoconstriction before any positive inotropic effect develops.
The drug is relatively poorly excreted in the elderly and should be given in smaller doses, otherwise there is a much increased risk of toxic effects. Digitoxin has a longer plasma half-life, and ouabain can only be given parenterally, with the same disadvantages as with intravenous digoxin; these drugs therefore have no place in the treatment of heart failure.

205.   A   Ref: 19,875
β-blockade produces improved ventricular filling, decreased out-flow tract gradients and a reduction in exercise-induced tachycardia. Atrial fibrillation is a serious development and should be dealt with promptly by electroversion followed by drug therapy to prevent recurrence. Verapamil may be effective when β-blockers have failed, and has been reported to reduce ventricular hypertrophy in some patients. Diuretics are given only for congestive heart failure. If atrial fibrillation becomes chronic, digitalis should be given to control the ventricular rate.

206.   A B C E   Ref: 19,877
In Hurler's syndrome heart failure is the cause of death in two-thirds of the patients, at an average age of 11 years. The heart is probably always abnormal in Friedreich's ataxia (ECG abnormalities in 90%) and at least half the cases die in heart failure.
In Duchenne muscular dystrophy heart failure is common; in limb girdle and facioscapulohumeral dystrophy it is rare. Pompe's disease is a glycogen storage disorder with massive glycogen deposition in all striated muscle, cardiac as well as skeletal; cardiac failure develops between 2 and 6 months of age.

207.   A B C   Ref: 19,864
The pain radiates to the shoulder but rarely to either arm. There is elevation of ST segments, maximum in lead II of the limb leads, without reciprocal depression in other leads. Pathological Q waves never occur.

208.   A B C E   Ref: 19,869
Pericardial effusion may develop in rheumatic fever but tamponade is unknown and aspiration is unnecessary. All the other conditions may cause tamponade.

209. **B C**   Ref: 19,862,863
Dissection involving the ascending aorta carries a high risk of rupture into the pericardium or severe aortic regurgitation, and surgery offers a better chance than medical treatment. The blood-pressure should be *reduced* by intravenous sodium nitroprusside, and because of the risks involved investigation must be pursued urgently.

210. **D E**   Ref: 19,896,897
In primary hyperaldosteronism the serum potassium is usually below 3.0 mmol/l; a level of 3.5 mmol/l might well be due to secondary aldosteronism, eg. in malignant hypertension, or to the use of diuretics. A raised serum uric acid is found in some 40% of patients with untreated essential hypertension. IVU is seldom helpful in unselected cases; it is reserved for patients under 40, diabetics with a pressure over 120 mmHg, patients whose pressure is diffult to control and patients suspected of having renal disease.

211. **A B D E**   Ref: 20,914
Vagal overactivity suggests *posterior* infarction. Occasionally in diabetic or in elderly patients pain may be absent.

212. **D E**   Ref: 20,914
The earliest change is ST elevation with reciprocal ST depression over the side opposite to the infarct. In transmural infarction pathological Q waves usually develop within the first 24 hours.

213. **A B C E**   Ref: 20,919
Treatment should combine inotropic agents with vasodilators such as sodium nitroprusside. The pulmonary venous congestion will probably require the administration of diuretics in large doses.

214. **A B C D E**   Ref: 20,922
A normal response involves a rise in heart rate to at least 120/min., without chest pain, significant dyspnoea or ECG changes.

215. **A ⊢ B**   Ref: 20,923,924
β-blockade with timolol or propranolol has been shown to reduce mortality. None of the other agents has been shown to have any definite effect. — *crap*
Aspirin is of definite benefit

216. **A B C E**   Ref: 20,908
There may be an S4 (atrial) or S3 (ventricular) gallop; the murmur of mitral insufficiency may become audible. The ECG may show ST depression.

217. **A B C E**   Ref: 20,911
The role of anticoagulants is uncertain; the evidence of benefit from their use in unstable angina is not convincing.   *Bed rest is the indication for heparin.*

218.   C E   Ref: 20,912

There is now general agreement that coronary artery spasm is not rare and that it may produce severe myocardial ischaemia progressing to infarction and death. β-blockers may aggravate coronary artery spasm and are best avoided. Surgery is reserved for those patients with continuing angina resistant to medical treatment.

219.   A B E   Ref: 20,948

The basic biochemical defect is unknown. The lungs at birth are physiologically normal.

220.   A B E   Ref: 20,U123,U124

Heterozygotes for α-antitrypsin deficiency have lower levels of activity of the enzyme than normals but their pulmonary function is normal; only among homozygotes does the characteristic clinical abnormality develop. There is no longer significant atmospheric pollution in cities and the correlation between air pollution and chest disease has disappeared. Wood workers have an increased incidence of adeno-carcinoma of their nasal sinuses and the same is true of shoe makers.

221.   B C E   Ref; 20,927,929

Any condition which shortens the thoracic spine will give an increased PA diameter of the chest. Hyperresonance is a very unreliable indication.

222.   A B D E   Ref: 20,938,939

In restrictive lung disease there is often a low PEF combined with a low TLC.

223.   A B C D   Ref: 20,940

The first four items are all examples of Type I respiratory failure, in which the hypoxaemia is accompanied by hyperventilation. In chronic bronchitis with emphysema (an example of Type II respiratory failure) there is inadequate ventilation and the PCO_2 is raised.

224.   D E   Ref: 21,969

There is seldom any need for oxygen if the Pa_2 is 60mm/h or above, and no need to raise it above this level by therapy. Oral analeptics are of no avail when given orally as long-term therapy, and all (including doxapram) are toxic if given in excessive dosage.

Venesection may be helpful if secondary polycythaemia is present.

225.   All false   Ref: 21,991

Radiotherapy may provide valuable palliation for specific symptoms but does not prolong survival.

226. **A C D E**   Ref: 21,992,993
Combinations of three of four drugs are more effective than single-drug regimes.

227. **B C**   Ref: 21,965
The disease affects children and young adults. Cyanosis is a characteristic sign. No really effective treatment is known but anticoagulants are often used.

228. **A D E**   Ref: 21,978
Infection via cow's milk has been virtually eliminated. The small respiratory droplets are not held back by gauze masks.
The tuberculin reaction becomes positive in 3 to 6 weeks after primary infection. Some organisms always enter the blood stream; usually this produces no clinical result but in a few cases miliary tuberculosis develops.

229. **A B C E**   Ref: 21,980
Anergy may follow measles, not varicella.

230. **A B D E**   Ref: 21,980-982
Ethambutol is bacteriostatic.

231. **B E**   Ref: 21,983
The nodes are typically *not* tender. Chemotherapy should be for 18 months. Surgery does not improve the results and may encourage sinus formation.

232. **A C**   Ref: 21,U125-127
Occasional strains resistant to penicillin have been described.
Bacteriological diagnosis can be made by detection of pneumococcal antigen in sputum by countercurrent immuno-electrophoresis.
Complete X-ray resolution can take up to 6 weeks.

233. **C D E**   Ref: 21,U126,U127
Klebsiella pneumonia should be treated with gentamicin and a cephalosporin, and legionnaires' disease with erythromycin.

234. **E**   Ref: 22,1016,1017
The characteristic findings on auscultation are crackles; wheezes suggest an element of bronchial obstruction, which is not normally present. Similarly the characteristic pattern of lung function tests is restrictive, not obstructive. The $PaCO_2$ is kept normal, or even lowered, by hyperventilation. Symptoms develop within 4 to 8 hours of exposure.

235. **B D E**   Ref: 22,1016,1017
Farmers' lung is a response to products of thermophilic actinomycetes which have grown in stored hay; the peak incidence in the UK is from

January to March. The characteristic chest X-ray changes of allergic alveolitis have not been seen in patients with humidifier fever. The antigen particle size must be less than $10\mu m$ for it to reach the respiratory bronchiole.

236.   A C E   Ref: 22,1004,1005

Reversibility does not distinguish asthma from the other forms of airways obstruction; the response may be absent in asthma, and may vary greatly in an individual patient from time to time.
Desensitization to specific allergens plays only a small part in management. The effect of sodium cromoglycate is preventive; it should not be used to treat an exacerbation.

237.   E   Ref:22,999

Many asthmatic children wheeze in the first 1 - 2 years of life, but few of these develop troublesome asthma. Persistence into adult life depends on the severity of the illness in childhood; of those with trivial asthma about half stop wheezing in early adolescence, but nearly all with chronic asthma continue to wheeze into adult life. Delayed puberty is common in chronic asthma but permanent growth retardation is very rare.

238.   A   Ref: 22,1000

A chest X-ray is essential to exclude other causes of bronchial obstruction. The remaining tests are seldom helpful.

239.   A C D E   Ref: 22,1012

The first lesion usually appears in an upper zone.

240.   A C D E   Ref: 22,1042

Retinal phakomas occur in tuberous sclerosis.

241.
         B   Ref: 22,1030,1031

The acute onset with erythema nodosum and hilar lymphadenopathy suggests a benign self-limiting course, whereas an insidious onset is likely to be associated with progressive organ damage.
The SACE test is positive in 60% of cases of sarcoid but it is also positive in other disorders mimicking sarcoid and is therefore unreliable. The disease is commoner in blacks than in whites, with a greater tendency to skin, joint and eye involvement. HLA testing has been inconclusive but the increased incidence in siblings compared with spouses suggests that some hereditary factor exists.

242.   B C D   Ref: 22,1020.1021

The defect is a restrictive one and both FVC and FEV_1 are reduced. The Pa CO_2 is characteristically *low*.

243. C   Ref: 22,1023
The best that can be hoped for from steroid therapy is some alleviation. Chest X-ray apppearances and lung function tests correlate poorly with clinical progress. Immunosuppressive drugs should be used as steroid-sparing agents. Penicillamine is thought to have helped some younger patients but is not generally indicated. Younger patients and women live longer.

244. C E   Ref: 22,1043,1044
Eosinophilia occurs in less than 30% of cases. Cysts very seldom calcify unless they are dead. Fever occurs in 20% of patients with solitary cysts and 44% of those with multiple cysts.

245. A B C E   Ref: 22,1038
Cholesterol crystals are seen in certain chronic effusions which are often of unknown cause. In obstruction of the thoracic duct the effusion is chylous, i.e. it is milky in appearance and contains fat globules.

246. A B C E   Ref: 22,1045
The eosinophilia is usually greater than 1×10^9 /1. 80% of the cases of pulmonary eosinophilia seen in the U.K. are due to this cause. There is no tissue invasion and mycotic abscesses (lung, kidneys, brain) are a feature of scepticaemic aspergillosis (Type III). The delayed (4-10 hours) haemorrhagic Arthus reponse is seen in up to 80% of Type II cases but in only 3% of asthmatics.

247. A C D   Ref: 22,1014,1015
Wheezes are uncommon compared with crackles; they indicate the presence of airway obstruction. Lung cancer is nine times commoner than in the general population. Treatment is symptomatic; steroids are of no value.

248. A C E   Ref: 22.1015
The increased hazard from cigarette smoking is that of lung cancer (90 times that of the non-exposed non-smoker). No effective therapy exists. Biopsy is needed for the diagnosis but there is a risk of tumour growth in the needle track or thoracotomy wound.

249. A D E   Ref: 25,1163,1164
HbF has the constitution of $\alpha_2 \gamma_2$. Raised levels of HbF occur in many unrelated anaemias and haemoglobinopathies in adults.

250. B E   Ref: 25,1173
In β-thalassaemia major splenomegaly may cause hypersplenism with increased transfusion requirements; in such a situation splenectomy is beneficial. Deletion of all four α genes leads to hydrops fetalis and stillbirth. Iron should only be given if there is clear evidence of iron deficiency.

251.   **B**   Ref: 25,1173
Except in the Hb Bart's-hydrops fetalis syndrome, fetoscopy with sampling
of fetal blood is necessary; the fetal mortality even in expert hands is 5 -
10%. To diagnose Hb Bart's hydrops fetalis amniocentesis is sufficient and
is justified if abortion to anticipate stillbirth is required. If both parents have
β-thalassaemia minor there is a 1 in 4 chance of the child having β-
thalassaemia major and an attempt at antenatal diagnosis would be
warranted if the parents understood the risks of the procedure and were not
prepared to accept the possibility of a severely affected child. Hb-H disease
is compatible with nearly normal life and fetoscopy would be unjustifiable.

252.   **A B C**   Ref: 25,1150,1151
The addition of iron to protoporphyrin converts it to haem.
Transferrin is the glycoprotein transport molecule for iron; it combines with
iron but normally some two-thirds of the serum transferrin are uncombined;
thus iron is not an *essential* component of transferrin.

253.   **A D**   Ref: 25,1154
A serum ferritin level below $15\mu g/1$ (normal $14\text{-}400\mu g/1$) is an infallible
indication of iron deficiency since it reflects depletion of the soluble
intracellular iron stores. MCHC and MCH are indices of microcytosis
rather than iron deficiency and are reduced in thalassaemia, sideroblastic
anaemia and the anaemia of chronic disease. Free erythrocyte protoporphyrin
represents porphyrin rings for which no iron is available for conversion to
haem. Its concentration rises early in iron deficiency, but this change is not
specific as it also occurs in lead poisoning, sideroblastic anaemia and
erythropoietic protoporphyria.

254.   **A C D E**   Ref: 25,1182,1183
The most reliable indices of early DIC are those which detect conversion of
fibrinogen to fibrin. The ethanol gelation and protamine sulphate precipitation
tests detect fibrin molecules which have not yet become involved in clot
formation. Fibrin degeneration products can be measured directly, and by
their interference with the action of thrombin on fibrinogen will prolong the
thrombin clotting time. The prothrombin time is prolonged in more severe
DIC.

255.   **A B C E**   Ref: 25,1172,1186,1189
Alcohol has a direct toxic effect on the marrow cells; this disappears within
a few days of alcohol withdrawal. Gluten-sensitive enteropathy causes
folate deficiency. β-thalassaemia trait characteristically leads to the
production of red cells that are *smaller* than normal.

256.   **D E**   Ref: 25,1188
Patients with a family history of PA or thyroid disease tend to present at a
younger age. About half the patients have intrinsic factor antibodies but

only about one-third have a family history.
Because of the gastric achlorhydra peptic ulcer is unknown, but there is a risk of gastric cancer.

257. A C D E   Ref: 25,1187,1188
The serum folate level quoted is within normal limits and this is consistent with PA. 200 ng of B_{12} represents 20% of a dose of $1\mu g$ and this is well within normal limits; intestinal absorption is normal and PA is excluded. Plasma radioactivity normally exceeds 0.6% of the oral dose per litre of plasma. Failure of response may be due to a second condition which has been overlooked, such as folate deficiency or gastric carcinoma.

258. A B D E   Ref: 25,1190
The RE system is well repleted with iron and it is thought that a failure to *release* iron from RE stores plays a part.

259. A D E   Ref: 25,1191
Sideroblastic anaemia may be caused by chronic *lead* poisoning.

260. D   Ref: 25,1176,1179
Aspirin interferes with platelet function and may precipitate episodes of bleeding in a haemophiliac. Haemotomas should be treated with rest and factor replacement and will then usually resolve quickly without surgery. Factor levels of 30% are suitable to control a haemarthrosis but for surgery 100% should be aimed at. Hepatitis remains a problem even with modern preparations.

261. B D E   Ref: 25,1798,1180
All the daughters of a haemophiliac must be carriers. A carrier has a 1 in 4 chance of producing a carrier daughter at each pregnancy.

262. A D   Ref: 26,1226
Methotrexate is widely used in the long-term treatment of acute leukaemia. Its use in patients with psoriasis has been associated with liver cirrhosis; otherwise liver function is unaffected. When high doses are being given, with 'planned rescue' by folinic acid, the delay in excretion caused by slow release of the drug from ascites or pleural effusions may prolong exposure to dangerous blood levels and cause acute toxic effects.

263. B C D E   Ref: 26,1239
Thrombocytopenia is a common manifestation of SLE, not of polyarteritis. Any cause of splenomegaly, eg. portal cirrhosis, may lead to a fall in platelet count through increased splenic sequestration. Massive transfusion produces the effect by dilution, Gram-negative septicaemia by increased consumption and chloramphenicol as a result of bone-marrow aplasia.

264.   **B C E**   Ref: 26,1239.
Platelets have an active metabolism and need to carry out both aerobic and anaerobic glycolysis for normal function. Intra-cranial haemorrhage is unlikely if the count is over 20 x $10^9/1$ (provided platelet function is normal).

265.   **A B C E**   Ref: 26,1242
For the first transfusion, cells from donors unmatched for HLA antigens may be used; a reaction is unlikely. However for repeated transfusions donors who are HLA-compatible must be found.

266.   **A**   Ref: 26,1229
About 20% of patients with BMG will develop a plasma-cell or lymphocytic neoplasm within 10 years. The patients are not anaemic, and clinically are in normal health. The finding of any plasma-cell tumour, whether in soft tissue or in bone, means that the process is no longer benign and that the diagnosis is incorrect.

267.   **A B C D E**   Ref: 26,1230
Epistaxis and retinal haemorrhage are two manifestations of the general bleeding tendency in this condition. Increased blood viscosity accounts for a variety of neurological phenomena including vertigo and nystagmus.

268.   **A C E**   Ref: 26,1201
Methotrexate blocks folate metabolism and this is the cause of the megaloblastic anaemia. Corticosteroids cause a fall in circulating T-lymphocytes and an impairment of cell-mediated, rather than humoral, immunity.

269.   **A D E**   Ref: 26,1202,1203
Raised lactic dehydrogenase and reduced or absent haptoglobin are non-specific and may occur in both intravascular and extra-vascular haemolysis. Intravascular haemolysis causes excretion of haemoglobin from the plasma via the kidneys, where tubular cells take it up, destroy it and store its iron; later these cells are shed and haemosiderin can be demonstrated in the sediment by the Prussian blue reaction. Favism causes intravascular haemolysis.

270.   **A**   Ref: 26,1209,1210
Meningeal leukaemia may develop during haematological remission and occurs in 5-10% of children with acute leukaemia even after prophylaxis with intrathecal methotrexate and cranial irradiation. In treatment, methotrexate is given *intrathecally;* if cranial irradiation has already been given, the benefit of further irradiation is problematic as there is a risk of leukoencephalopathy if more is given.

271. **B C D**   Ref: 26,1196,1197
Sparing of neutrophils is not uncommon at presentation; the cells may show
toxic granulation and increased alkaline phosphatase activity. Bone marrow
aspirate is essential to make sure that no abnormal cells are present but
trephine biopsy gives a better indication of marrow cellularity. Reticulin
staining of trephine samples may help in excluding myeloproliferative or
preleukaemic disorders. Extramedullary haemopoiesis is absent in aplastic
anaemia.

272. **B C**   Ref: 26,1214,1216
The prognosis in Philadelphia-negative CGL is worse; such patients often
fail to respond to busulphan or hydroxyurea, which are nearly always
effective in Ph-positive patients. The Ph chromosome may occur in some
lymphocytes. Its presence is not related to the low neutrophil alkaline
phosphatase.

273. **B C E**   Ref: 23,1067,1068
The haematuria of schistosomiasis is due to bleeding from the bladder and
typically occurs at the end of micturition. Bleeding from the glomeruli is
often brownish or 'smoky' in appearance.

274. **E**   Ref: 23,1049,1050
Plasma creatinine levels are unaffected by prolonged tourniquet time or by
anticoagulants and the rise with meat ingestion or aspirin therapy is trivial.
Some patients with quite advanced renal failure have augmented renal
tubular secretion of creatinine which may result in their plasma creatinine
levels being much lower than would be expected.

275. **A B C E**   Ref: 23,1090
Recent tuberculosis or cancer, and chronic suppurative disease, are
indications for dialysis rather than transplantation; in the presence of
osteodystrophy transplantation is preferable.

276. **C D E**   Ref: 23,1091,1092
The daily protein intake should be 1.25 - 1.5g/kg/day, otherwise muscle
wasting will occur. No salt restriction is necessary unless it is needed to
control hypertension. All dialysis patients are anaemic and so while
moderate exercise may be beneficial, strenuous exertion is impossible. Tap
water often contains small amounts of aluminium and this may accumulate
and cause toxic effects, (severe osteomalacia, dialysis dementia).

277. **A D E**   Ref: 23,1094
Original diabetes or analgesic nephropathy are unfavourable.
Third-party blood transfusion gives an increase of 20-30% in graft success
rate.

278. **B D E** Ref: 23,1086-1088
Co-trimoxazole may cause permanent deterioration of glomerular filtration rate. Mild hyperlipidaemia is common in chronic renal failure, but there is no evidence that dietary or drug therapy aimed at lowering lipid levels is beneficial (unless the levels are very high).

279. **A B C E** Ref: 23,1054,1055
In patients with myeloma, urography may cause precipitation of protein within the tubules. The urine should be rendered alkaline and adequate hydration ensured beforehand. The role of steroids in preventing severe reactions is still uncertain.

280. **A B C D** Ref: 23,1064
Exposure to cold in susceptible subjects may produce haemoglobinuria, not haematuria.

281. **A C** Ref: 23,1064,1065
Pruritus may be a presenting feature. Anaemia is almost invariable in chronic renal failure and by no means indicates a terminal state.

282. **A C** Ref: 23,1076,1077
There is loss of blood from lungs and kidney, and anaemia is always present. Cyclophosphamide is given in conjunction with plasma exchange. Without treatment the condition is uniformly fatal but with plasma exchange some 60% of patients may be expected to survive.

283. **A E** Ref: 23,1072,1073
The relapse rate is very high, particularly in children. About 90% of children, but only about 60% of adults, respond to prednisolone.

284. **B C D E** Ref: 23,1080
Plasmodium malariae causes quartan malaria, in which renal complications are very rare. The danger arises from *P. falciparum* infection (malignant tertian) in which blackwater fever may develop with massive intravascular haemolysis. Sickle-cell disease and typhoid fever may also act in this way and in the latter there may also be disseminated intravascular coagulation. *Schistosoma haematobium* infection may cause obstructive uropathy and in leptospirosis acute tubulo-interstitial nephritis may develop.

285. **B C E** Ref: 23,1079,1081
For a 70 kg patient a urine volume of 400 ml/day suffices for adequate excretion. A urine/plasma osmolality of less than 1.1 suggests ATN, as does a urine sodium of over 20 mmol/l. A urine urea of 200 mmol/l implies urine/plasma ratio of about 10 which makes ATN unlikely.

286. **B E** Ref:24,1114
The association with nerve deafness is not invariable. Inheritance is

135

autosomal dominant with varying penetrance. Antenatal diagnosis is not possible.

287. **A C D**   Ref: 24,1115
Although clinical hepatic disease is not seen, in one-third of the patients there are clusters of dilated bile-ducts. About 10% of patients have aneurysms of the cerebral arteries and these may rupture. There is no evidence of an increased risk of malignancy.

288. **B C D**   Ref: 24,1114-6,1118
In Finnish congenital nephrotic syndrome about 80% die from persistent infections in the first year of life. Familial recurrent haematuria is a benign condition.

289. **A B D E**   Ref:24,1139,1140
Budd-Chiari syndrome may result from growth of the tumour into the inferior vena cava and the hepatic vein. Hypertension may be a consequence of Wilm's tumour. Hypercalcaemia may be due either to bony metastases or to ectopic production.

290. **A C**   Ref: 24,1110,1111,1113
Uric acid and cystine are more soluble in alkaline media but the pH makes little difference to the solubility of calcium oxalate, and triple phosphate stones are nearly always formed in alkaline urine (often in the presence of urea-splitting organisms).
Methionine stones do not occur.

291. **B D**   Ref: 24,1111
There is some evidence that the incidence of oxalate stones is *lower* in hard water areas. A high intake of ascorbic acid will *increase* the urinary excretion of oxalate. A milk-free diet reduces phosphate intake and hence the urinary excretion of pyrophosphate; the latter is thought to have a protective action against the precipitation of calcium oxalate.

292. **B C**   Ref: 24,1142,1143,1145
In mixed connective tissue disease biopsy, if abnormal, it is likely to show a non-specific picture of diffuse proliferative or membranous nephritis. The demonstration of mesangial IgA is diagnostic of H-S purpura. In thrombotic thrombocytopenic purpura (Moschowitz's syndrome) biopsy is absolutely contra-indicated because of the coagulation defect. The Churg-Strauss variety of polyarteritis, with asthma and eosinophilia, rarely affects the kidney.

293. **A B**   Ref: 24,1142,1143,1145
Steroids and immunosuppressants are ineffective in C,D & E but attacks of

familial Mediterranean fever can often be reduced or prevented by the administration of colchicine.

294. **A C D**   Ref: 24,1146
Urate crystals are deposited in the medullary interstitium, the pyramids and the papilae. Pyuria and haematuria are uncommon unless renal stones and infection are present.

295. **A C D**   Ref: 24,1106,1107
Useful films may still be obtained with a blood-urea over 16 mmol/l if a high dose of contrast is given and tomography is carried out. The prostatic impression on the bladder is quite unreliable as a guide to the size of the gland.

296. **A D E**   Ref: 24,1109
A raised ESR is typical. There is some evidence that corti-costeroids are beneficial in idiopathic cases.

297. **A D E**   Ref: 24,1132,1134,1136
The excretion route for aspirin is primarily renal and reduced doses are necessary. Codeine and morphine are excreted by the liver and may safely be used in renal failure. Colchicine should not be given on a long-term basis to renal failure patients. The excretion route for most β-blocking drugs is hepatic, but for atenolol it is renal; the use of this drug in renal failure is dangerous.

298. **B C E**   Ref: 24,1130-1134
Drugs B, C & E are significantly removed by dialysis; drugs A & D are not.

299. **B C D E**   Ref: 24,1127,1128
Paracetamol alone in therapeutic dosage does not cause renal damage, but if it or phenacetin is combined with aspirin, protection against oxidative damage to the renal tubules is removed.

300. **B D**   Ref: 24,1097.1098
The demonstration of covert bacteriuria in a pregnant women implies a high risk of acute pyelonephritis later in pregnancy.
Screening of all women attending antenatal clinics should be carried out and patients showing covert bacteriuria should be given appropriate chemotherapy. Chronic prostatitis in males may be a cause of covert bacteriuria. Urea-splitting organisms may raise the pH of the urine and contribute to the formation of triple phosphate stones. In the urethral syndrome, bacteriuria, if present, is by definition not covert. Ordinary bacteriology shows no infection; special techniques give positive results in some cases but a residue remains in which no bacteria can be shown.

301.   **A B**   Ref: 24,1099,1100

Analgesic nephropathy may give IVU appearances similar to those of reflux nephropathy but the two only rarely occur together.

There is seldom any point in surgery to correct the reflux; the damage has already been done in childhood and treatment should concentrate on the prevention and treatment of urinary infection and hypertension. Many patients are salt-losers and will require *supplements* of dietary salt.

302.   **A C D**   Ref: 24,1101,1103

Although UTI is commoner in females throughout most of childhood, the sex ratio is reversed in the first few months. The younger the child, the more susceptible are the kidneys to permanent damage from UTI. Acidosis raises the possibility of obstruction which requires urgent investigation and treatment. VUR is by far the most important cause of renal scarring but P-fimbriated strains of E.coli may be able to ascend the urinary tract in the absence of VUR.

303.   **B C E**   Ref: 27,1276,1278

Solar elastosis is a synonym for chronic benign actinic damage to the skin. Seborrhoeic keratosis may resemble solar keratosis but it is benign.

304.   **B D E**   Ref: 27,1245

Koebner's phenomenon is the development of the lesions of the skin disease concerned along scratch-marks; it is well recognized in psoriasis, lichen planus and warts.

305.   **A B C D E**   Ref: 27,1275

All are correct.

306.   **C D E**   Ref: 27,1251

Clobetasol is one of the more potent steroids, and while all topical steroids are absorbed to some extent, the risk is higher with the more active drugs. There is a risk when topical steroids are used on the face of precipitating perioral eczema or rosacea, but they are very effective in treating eczema or discoid lupus erythematosus. If the wrong vehicle is used for dilution, serious loss of potency may occur. Skin sensitivity may develop to preservatives added to the base.

307.   **A B D E**   Ref: 27,1285,1286

Both ethinyloestradiol and cyproterone shift the oestrogen-androgen balance in favour of the former. Retinoic acid (topical) or 13-cis-retinoic acid (oral) are effective; they are *derivatives* of vitamin A. Oral prednisone may be given with ethinyloestradiol and helps to suppress adrenal androgen production. Co-trimoxazole is effective in controlling the bacterial element in the disease.

308. **B**   Ref: 27,1279,1280

Metastasis is so rare that it should prompt a review of the diagnosis. The incidence is equal in the two sexes. Radiotherapy is an accepted mode of treatment. The prognosis is excellent, with a 5-year survival of 99%.

309. **A C D**   Ref: 27,1280,1281

Origin from a pre-existing mole can be inferred with certainty in only 50% of patients. Excision is the preferred treatment; cryosurgery is at present experimental.

310. **B D E**   Ref: 27,1266

There is no strong association with any HLA type. The disease may appear at any age. Guttate psoriasis may be precipitated by an infection with *Strep. pyogenes.*

311. **A C D**   Ref: 27,1270

PUVA is thought to increase the risk of skin cancer. Toxicity of psoralens in combination with UVA is restricted to the skin and the eyes.

312. **B C E**   Ref: 27,1264

Carbonless copy paper may act as an irritant to the facial mucous membranes. Industrial cutting fluids are oil-in-water emulsions and these too act as irritants.

313. **A B D**   Ref: 28,1325,1327

Bullous impetigo is almost invariably staphylococcal. Kaposi's varicelliform eruption is a synonym for eczema herpeticum, a severe infection with herpes simplex in a subject with defective immunity or with atopic eczema.

314. **A B D E**   Ref: 28,1327

The mortality of neonatal herpes simplex is 50%. Genital herpes may be caused by either Type 1 of Type 2 virus.

315. **A B C E**   Ref: 28,1307,1308

Pressure urticaria responds poorly to antihistamines; in exceptionally severe cases oral steroid therapy may be effective.

For urticarial vasculitis the most effective treatment is with steroids, but antihistamines often help to relieve the symptoms.

316. **B D**   Ref: 28,1333,1334

The commonest cause is *Ankylostoma braziliense,* but other hookworms and *Strongyloides spp.* (including *S. stercoralis*) may less commonly be responsible. The disease is self-limiting. In severe infestations there may be pulmonary infiltration and marked eosinophilia (Loeffler's syndrome). Thioganine is a cytostatic drug used in the treatment of acute myeloblastic leukaemia; the drug of choice in cutaneous larva migrans is thiabendazole.

317. **A E** Ref: 28,1320
About 85% of patients have HLA B8/DRw3. Although the patient usually describes the occurrence of blisters, these have nearly always been ruptured by scratching by the time he is examined.
The response to dapsone is so reliable that a trial of the drug is often recommended as a diagnostic test.

318. **A C E** Ref: 29,1371,1374
The pupil is small and reacts poorly. Keratic precipitates are masses of inflammatory cells and debris which become deposited on the lens and posterior surface on the cornea. The course is usually short (3-6 weeks) but the condition tends to recur.

319. **A B C D** Ref: 29,1385,1386
Cryptococcal eye infection occurs more often in the absence of immunosuppression and usually involves the optic nerve head.

320. **A C D** Ref: 29,1378,1379
Glaucoma is three times commoner in blacks than in whites. The most important diagnostic features are cupping of the optic disc and loss of peripheral vision; intra-ocular pressure measurements are variable and of limited value.

321. **A D** Ref: 29,1346
Local drops are often ineffective even in the presence of a perforation, and in any case may be difficult to instil in a young child. Cholesteatoma is not uncommon and should always be kept in mind in children with otitis. The adenoids should only be removed when they are demonstrably enlarged.

322. **A C D** Ref: 29,1347,1348
A positive Rinne test in a deaf ear indicates sensorineural deafness; the defect in chronic otitis media and in tympanosclerosis is conductive and in these the Rinne test would be expected to be negative (bone conduction better than air conduction).

323. **A B E** Ref: 29,1369,1370
The phenotype of 47,XXY is Klinefelter's syndrome, which is not associated with cataract. However, some trisomy conditions (trisomy 21, Down's syndrome; trisomy 13, Patau's syndrome; and trisomy 18, Edward's syndrome) are so associated. Hypocalcaemia, not hypercalcaemia, is associated with cataract.

324. **A E** Ref: 29,1366,1368
Besides photophobia there is intense spontaneous pain. Light shone into the sound eye will cause contraction of the pupil in the affected eye and this is painful in iritis and glaucoma but not in corneal ulceration. Flare (scattered

light from a beam shone in the eye) is due to the presence of inflammatory cells in the aqueous humour and is a manifestation of uveitis.

325. **A B** Ref: 29,1364,1365
CT scanning is particularly valuable in determining the intracranial extent, if any, of a meningioma, ultrasound is unable to penetrate the bony boundary of the skull. For the outlining of cystic lesions however, ultrasound is superior. Lymphomas and lacrimal gland tumours can be identified by either technique.

326. **A C E** Ref: 29,1341,1342
The accumulation is composed of keratin, not cholesterol. Mastoidectomy is often *required* to prevent its recurrence.

327. **E** Ref: 29,1353
Muco-purulent discharge only develops in the presence of infection.
Desensitization is of limited value and may cause anaphylaxis.
Topical steroids are valuable and have no systemic effects.
Sodium cromoglycate is often effective if used for prevention rather than treatment. Most antihistamines have a marked sedative effect.

328. **A B D E** Ref: 29,1383,1384
There is no convincing evidence that correction before 6 months is superior but correction after 2 years is certainly much less effective.

329. **A D** Ref: 29,1342,1343
Tinnitus may be caused by abnormalities in the external, middle or inner ear. At least half of all patients with tinnitus have essentially normal hearing. The sex incidence is roughly equal.
Anti-depressants may help a depressed patient to ignore the tinnitus but do not alter its intensity.

330. **B D E** Ref: 30,1415,1416
The concept of concussion as a functional disturbance without structural brain damage is no longer thought to be tenable; injuries associated with even brief unconsciousness probably cause some degree of physical damage. Fatal brain damage can occur without any scalp injury or skull fracture.

331. **A C D** Ref: 30,417,1418
Only a good quality skull radiograph can exclude a fracture.
About 5% of patients admitted with a head injury have a fit in the first week.

332. **B D E** Ref: 30,1421
Late epilepsy occurs in only about 5% of those admitted with head injury; about half of these have fits with a focal component.

333. **A C E** Ref: 30,1418,1419,1422
One third of patients with head injuries who die in hospital have talked following the injury. Some degree of dehydration reduces the risk of brain oedema, so intravenous fluids should not be given unless injuries elsewhere have caused hypovolaemic shock.

334. **C E** Ref: 30,1395
The organic nature of Alzheimer's disease is evident at an early stage from certain primitive reflexes which appear: sucking and pouting, glabella tap, tonic grasp and palmomental. Motor apraxia also develops early. Insight is often retained at first and this leads to depression. On the other hand a spastic weakness affecting one leg only is inconsistent with the diffuse atrophy of the disease.

335. **A C D E** Ref: 30,1398
Ice-cold water should not be used; it causes vasoconstriction and shivering which conserve the core temperature.

336. **B C D** Ref: 30,1401
Clonic hand movements may occur in petit mal; the condition remits by early adult life.

337. **A B D** Ref: 30,1412,1413
Phenobarbitone may cause skin rashes or hirsutism. The hydantoins cause enzyme induction and more rapid inactivation of many drugs including oral contraceptives so the dose should be increased.

338. **A B D** Ref: 30,1410,1413
Intramuscular phenobarbitone is unsatisfactory as it is slow-acting and gives unstable levels of circulating drug. Tricyclic anti-depressants do not control epilepsy and may in fact provoke it.

339. **A D E** Ref: 30,1412,1413
Petit mal absences with grand mal seizures may respond to sodium valproate or to phenytoin. Acne may follow the use of barbiturates and hydantoins. Sodium valproate is teratogenic in animals and is not recommended in pregnancy.

340. **A B E** Ref: 30,1392
The pain lasts 15 minutes to 2 hours and there is no family history.

341. **A C E** Ref: 30,1393
If the diagnosis is clinically obvious treatment should be started at once without waiting for the biopsy result. Oculomotor palsies can result from occlusion of arteries in the orbit supplying the nerves and muscles concerned.

342. **B D E**   Ref: 30,1423,1426
After ulnar nerve transposition at the elbow there may be severe pain,
probably due to impairment of blood supply to the nerve.
Modified trigeminal gangliolysis by means of glycerol injection appears to
give good pain relief without significant sensory loss.

343. **A C E**   Ref: 31,1448,1449
Rupture of cavernous sinus aneurysms is unusual whereas pressure on the
IIIrd, IVth and VIth cranial nerves and the carotid sympathetic plexus is a
common source of symptoms. Anterior communicating aneurysms nearly
always present with haemorrhage.

344. **C**   Ref: 31,1451,1453
A subarachnoid haemorrhage is usually followed by intense cerebral
vasoconstriction and attempts to lower the blood pressure may cause
cerebral infarction. If the CSF is not examined, meningitis may be missed.
Patients over 65 should be treated conservatively unless the aneurysm is on
the internal carotid, when the risks of surgery are much lower. Patients in the
last category of the question should normally have bilateral carotid
angiography performed.

345. **B C D**   Ref: 31,1458,1460
Pentazocine can cause vomiting and should be avoided. Histological
identification by biopsy is usually desirable but in a patient with a dominant
hemisphere tumour who is reasonably well and whose management would
not be influenced by the result of biopsy it is better to avoid the risk of
neurological deficit. EEG is of little use in diagnosing or locating
intracerebral tumours.

346. **B C D**   Ref: 31,1461,1462
Overproduction of CSF is a very uncommon cause; the ususal explanation
is obstruction at some point in the CSF circulation.
The birth of a child with hydrocephalus, spina bifida or anencephaly
increases the likelihood of subsequent children being affected.

347. **A B D**   Ref: 31,1462,1475
The meningitic infections causing hydrocephalus are those in which there is
an inflammatory exudate, hence viral meningitis is not a cause. Toxoplasmosis,
a protozoan infection , can cause meningal exudates; toxocariasis is due to
infection with a nematode and does not involve the meninges (though it
commonly invades the eye).

348. **A B C D E**   Ref: 31,1462
Hydrocephalus by definition involves enlargement of the ventricles.

349. **C E**   Ref: 31,1462
Skull circumference measurements have to be interpreted in terms of the

child's growth curve and general development. If the fontanelles close without relief of the hydrocephalus, small additional ('Wormian') bones may develop in the fontanelles and sutures. The finding of calcification would suggest toxoplasmosis or a tumour.

350. **A B C**   Ref: 31,1462
The main clinical features in adults are intellectual deterioration and signs of raised intracranial pressure; thinning of the skull vault is less obvious than in children and changes in the clinoid processes are more helpful. Subarachnoid haemorrhage can cause blockage of CSF circulation in exactly the same way as meningitic exudates.

351. **C D E**   Ref: 31,1463,1464
The results in adults are very good; in children there is often irreversible damage to the brain which the shunt cannot relieve.
Infection of the shunt may be insidious in onset and may even fail to cause a fever. Revision of shunts is inevitable in children, for the simple reason that the child is still growing so that the tube needs to be lengthened from time to time.

352. **A B D**   Ref: 31,1470,1473
A child with tuberculous meningitis who is unconscious may be so not because of the extent of the meningitis but because of obstructive hydrocephalus with grossly raised intracranial pressure. An acute encephalopathy may follow immunization with live viruses (measles, poliomyelitis) and with pertussis vaccine. Intracranial haemorrhage can follow violent shaking with no evidence of head injury. Lumbar puncture in the presence of greatly raised intracranial pressure (as with a cerebral abscess) may be fatal.

353. **C D**   Ref: 31,1481,1482
There can be no doubt that tabes is a manifestation of neurosyphilis but *T. pallidum* cannot be demonstrated in the spinal cord. In a patient who has no neurological abnormality and whose serum anti-body tests are normal, after an adequate course of treatment, lumbar puncture is probably unnecessary. Steroids are of no use in a Herxheimer reaction and may make meningovascular syphilis worse.

354. **A B D E**   Ref: 31,1435,1436
The symptoms of onset indicate a single site of involvement in 80% of patients.

355. **A B D E**   Ref: 31,1437
Indications of a severe outcome include onset with brain-stem or cerebellar lesions, onset after the age of 40 and disease which is progressive from the onset.

356. **A C D**   Ref: 31,1438,1439
Diets high in unsaturated fatty acids appear to reduce the severity and length of relapses.

357. **B D**   Ref: 32,1484,1485
Hypertrophy of calf muscles is a classical finding in Duchenne muscular dystrophy but may also occur in spinal muscular atrophy and in adult metabolic myopathies. In dystrophia myotonica of sufficient duration, the wasting may be sufficient to mask the myotonia. Deep reflexes are usually present or reduced.
Weakness following a meal suggests periodic paralysis.

358. **B E**   Ref: 32,1486,1487
Carcinoma-associated cases account for only 17% of the total, the remainder being 'uncomplicated' (66%) or associated with connective-tissue disease (17%). In long-standing 'uncomplicated' cases cardiac conduction defects may be found. Steroid therapy reinforced with immuno-suppression, is the standard form of treatment.

359. **A B D**   Ref: 32,1489
Fever is a relatively late sign; early manifestations include unstable blood pressure, cardiac arrhythmia, *hyper*ventilation and cyanosis.

360. **B C**   Ref: 32,1514
Axonal degeneration occurs in some 20% of patients and in these full recovery is impossible; however, persistent complete paralysis is rare. Corneal damage is very uncommon if corneal sensation is intact, and tarsorrhaphy is unnecessary. There is still considerable doubt about the effectiveness of treatment with steroids.

361. **A B D E**   Ref: 32,1523,1525
Parenteral thiamine is absolutely essential in Wernicke's encephalopathy and in delirium tremens. Alcoholic cerebellar degeneration does not respond to thiamine and causes permanent disability.

362. **A C D E**   Ref: 32,1526,1527
Lesions of the sensory visual system do not produce inequality of the pupils. Uhthoff's phenomenon is a deterioration of visual acuity resulting from a rise in body temperature; it is characteristic of demyelinating disease affecting the optic nerves.

363. **A B C**   Ref: 32,1498,1500
Compression by structures outside the cord itself usually affects the nerve roots first. Ependymoma is an intrinsic tumour of the cord and epidural abscess causes local pain and tenderness followed by the rapid onset of paraparesis.

364. **A B C D**   Ref: 32,1500
Light touch is preserved bilaterally.

365. **A B C D E**   Ref: 32,1499,1502
In a case of MND it is essential to exclude a high cervical lesion.
Acute transverse myelopathy resembles acute cord compression clinically
and the latter must be excluded. Myelography is always needed for the
diagnosis of intraspinal tumours.

366. **A B**   Ref: 32,1512
Neuropathy in carcinoma of the lung, uraemia and diabetes is predominantly
sensory.

367. **A B E**   Ref: 32,1519
Small amounts of alcohol give temporary relief. Propranolol is often helpful.

368. **D E**   Ref: 32,1516,1518
Levodopa relieves the symptoms but does not halt progression. There is no
association with HLA antigens. Dementia is characteristic of the later
stages.

369. **A C**   Ref: 32,1490,1491
The antibody is IgG; its titre is raised in 90% of patients with generalized
disease and in 70% of patients with ocular disease.
It is still detectable in many patients in clinical remission.

370. **A C E**   Ref: 32,1491
Ocular symptoms are usually asymmetrical. Emotional stress, pregnancy
and infection may cause exacerbations.

371. **A E**   Ref: 33,1542
Lithium is effective in both unipolar and bipolar forms, rather more so in the
latter. It can be given to elderly patients but the dose may have to be
reduced. Cholinergic side-effects are characteristic of the tricyclic anti-
depressants; lithium may cause tremor, polyuria and weight gain. Vomiting
and diarrhoea indicate dangerously high blood levels (over 2 mmol/l) which
may be fatal if the drug is not withdrawn.

372. **A B D E**   Ref: 33,1542
All have a relatively long half-life except viloxazine.

373. **A C D E**   Ref: 33,1546,1548
The diagnosis of schizophrenia rests entirely on the patient's behaviour,
mental state and history; no laboratory investigations can offer diagnostic
help.

374.   A C E   Ref: 33,1549   poor
Catatonic symptoms and a normal affective response imply a good
prognosis.

375.   B C E   Ref: 33,1561
Benzodiazepines and tricyclic antidepressants cause drowsiness but are not
commonly the cause of dreams and nightmares.

376.   A D E   Ref: 33,1544,1545
Behaviour therapy is the treatment of choice for chronic phobic anxiety.
Long-term treatment with benzodiazepines may cause trouble in the shape
of withdrawal symptoms when treatment is stopped.

377.   A B C E   Ref: 33,1551
The incidence is highest among those living in urban areas.

378.   C   Ref: 34,1594,1595
Parental discipline is usually good, sometimes too strict. About half the
cases may be expected to have abdominal pains in adult life.
Similar symptoms in another member of the family are not uncommon.
Minor tranquillizers may be used if there is a prominent element of anxiety.

379.   B E   Ref: 34,1595
Bladder control in normal children may not be established until the age of 4.

380.   A C E   Ref: 34,1596
Amnesia for an episode of night terrors is total. The attacks occur in slow
wave phase 4 sleep.

381.   A B E   Ref: 34,1582,1583
Doctors under 54 years of age are less likely to have I.H.D. than the general
population. There is no significant difference in schizophrenia rates for
doctors and non-doctors.

382.   C D   Ref: 34,1605
Only insomnia, poor memory and anxiety are benefited, and in long term
studies (cross-over at 6 months) only insomnia and poor memory were
improved.

383.   A D   Ref: 34,1617
Prognosis is better for disabling symptoms and not so good for those that can
be turned on or off as required.

384.   B C   Ref: 34,1587,1588
The MAO inhibitors are particularly useful in the control of phobic anxiety,
and are just as effective as the tricyclics in mild depression.

385. **A D E** Ref: 34,1588
β-blockers are effective in relieving the results of β-adrenergic stimulation such as palpitations, flushing, tremor.

386. **A D E** Ref: 35,1658
Episodes of apnoea lasting up to 122 minutes have been observed in the normal human fetus. Maternal food intake causes an increase in breathing movements.

387. **C D** Ref: 35,1640
In uncomplicated pregnancies there is no evidence that hospital admission confers any benefit. Delivery before 38 weeks greatly increases the risk of neonatal respiratory distress syndrome and if it can be delayed to 39 weeks the outlook is much improved.
Purified insulin is less likely to evoke antibody formation, hence the risk of fetal β-cell damage is reduced. Urinary glucose measurement is unreliable in assessing diabetic control but it gives a measure of the rate of dietary carbohydrate loss.

388. **A B** Ref: 35,1636,1637
Diethyl-stilboestrol causes abnormalities of the genital tract in the fetus and predisposes to later development of vaginal carcinoma in girls. Chlorambucil, being an alkylating agent, is highly teratogenic, but no deleterious effects have ever been reported from azathioprine in correct dosage. Phenylbutazone may cause fetal goitre but it is not teratogenic.

389. **C** Ref: 35,1652
The baby may appear well immediately after birth; signs usually develop within 1 - 2 hours. The chest X-ray appearances are suggestive but not pathognomonic. Treatment with surfactants has no effect and antibiotics are not indicated.

390. **A B C D E** Ref: 35,1643
Raised α serum-fetoprotein is by no means diagnostic of neural defect.

391. **A C D E** Ref: 35,1634
Patients who have undergone curative cardiac surgery are at no increased risk. The remaining conditions are all associated with increased maternal mortality and are grounds for avoiding pregnancy altogether.

392. **A B E** Ref: 35,1642
The risk of the child developing diabetes is thought to be between 1% and 5%. Mental retardation is uncommon. The blood levels of both calcium and magnesium may fall significantly during the first 3 days of life if the mother is being treated with insulin; this is thought to be due to delayed development of the baby's parathyroid function.

393. **A C E** Ref: 35,1661
Male sex and polyhydramnios are risk factors.

394. **A C D** Ref: 36,1683
Ataxia telangiectasia and Tay-Sachs disease show autosomal recessive inheritance.

395. **A B D E** Ref: 36,1691
Glucuronidation of paracetamol is reduced but compensatory sulphation allows elimination rates comparable to those of adults.

396. **B D E** Ref: 36,1705
Alimentary absorption is only slightly impaired, if at all.
Hepatic conjugation is usually unaltered.

397. **A B C D E** Ref: 36,1706
All the drugs quoted can cause confusion. All diuretics, not only frusemide, may do so.

398. **E** Ref: 36,1713
Macular degeneration is commoner among women and occurs earlier than in men. Unilateral involvement is commoner than bilateral.
Choroidal vessels proliferate and penetrate the pigment epithelium and cause the foveal receptor cells to atrophy. Exposure to ultra violet light is a cause of cataract but not of macular degeneration .

399. **B C D** Ref: 36,1713
Only about 5% of the cases admitted have hypothyroidism. The P CO_2 is usually low because of reduced CO^2 production.

400. **B D** Ref: 36,1721,1722
Some malabsorption of calcium is common in osteoporosis but the evidence that this is the cause is not convincing, and osteoporosis is in fact commoner in countries with a high dietary calcium. A low body weight is associated with a slightly higher risk of osteoporosis. There is no good evidence that oral calcium is beneficial.

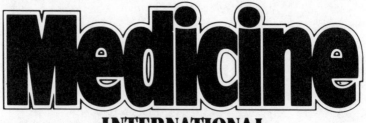

INTERNATIONAL